SpringerBriefs in Environmental Science

For further volumes:
http://www.springer.com/series/8868

Pankaj Gupta · Vijay Kumar Sharma
Sushma Sharma

Healing Traditions of the Northwestern Himalayas

Springer

Pankaj Gupta
Vijay Kumar Sharma
Institute of Integrated Himalayan Studies
Himachal Pradesh University
Shimla
Himachal Pradesh
India

Sushma Sharma
Department of Biosciences
Himachal Pradesh University
Shimla
Himachal Pradesh
India

ISSN 2191-5547 ISSN 2191-5555 (electronic)
ISBN 978-81-322-1924-8 ISBN 978-81-322-1925-5 (eBook)
DOI 10.1007/978-81-322-1925-5
Springer New Delhi Heidelberg New York Dordrecht London

Library of Congress Control Number: 2014940152

Printed on acid-free paper

Springer is part of Springer Science+Business Media (www.springer.com)

Dedicated to our most revered and beloved parents

Preface

Maintaining good health by making use of traditional curative techniques and using herbs is as old as the history of humanity. Traditional health care systems originated much before the evolution of modern medicines. Today, the world is looking back at the alternative system of medicine, because it attempts to examine and cure the cause of a disease, covering up all its symptoms. In the recent years, the use of the alternative system of medicine has got wider consideration and appreciation throughout the world. In some Asian and African countries, 80 % of the population depend on traditional medicine for primary health care. The book precisely unveils indigenous healthcare traditions among Himalayan communities besides delineating the conventional and conservative interventions made by people for both physical and mental health at the local level.The Himalayas has a rich legacy of folk medicine and other traditional healthcare practices. Besides *Ayurveda*, a number of ethnic healthcare systems remain widespread in the Himalayas.

The endeavor to maintain an optimum state of health has always exercised the mind of man, since time immemorial, which resulted in the evolution of diverse systems of healing across the world. Chapter 1 talks about the legacy of the Himalayan region, its people, their knowledge resources, and concept of healing in epic sagas.

The concept of health, categorization of healing traditions, folk medicine, and research studies on healing traditions carried out in the Himalayan region are presented in Chap. 2.

The thought of food as medicament and culinary traditions of the northwest Himalayas, are discussed in Chap. 3. This chapter also highlights the culinary customs of Himalayan communities with respect to its ethnic food, diversity, and suitability of food according to climatic conditions, ingredients used, and use of indigenous cookery technologies.

Chapter 4 is focused on mystic healers of the Himalayan region, who act as mediators between the materialistic and metaphysical world. The role of village deities and numerous Hindu Gods and Goddesses in healing is also discussed in this chapter. Sacred healing by Buddhist monks and use of plants in magico-religious ritualistic performances is incorporated in Chap. 4.

Mountain communities are dependent on forests for their livelihood and sustenance. They collect herbs for their own use and sale in the market. The process involved in collection of herbs, their processing, and their cultivation is taken up in Chap. 5. Traditional methods employed for preparing herbal formulations, dosage system, administering of medicine, traditional therapeutic procedures, pediatric medicine, indigenous dermatology, and cosmetology are also discussed this chapter. The role of traditional orthopedic practitioners, traditional birth attendants, and *Amchis* is taken up in this chapter.

Indigenous *Materia-Medica* is considered in Chap. 6. This includes the material used by folk herbalists in their medicines.

The healing traditions are on the verge of extinction, thus, an endeavor has been made to explore the reasons behind the fading of these systems into oblivion. The folk healers, herbalists, traditional birth attendants, orthopedic practitioners, oracles, shamans, and priests, who have shared their lifetime experience, are duly acknowledged for their cooperation. In addition to this I acknowledge the Director, Institute of Integrated Himalayan Studies, Himachal Pradesh University, Shimla and other members of the staff for their help & support. Every possible effort has been made while gathering and interpreting the information, yet the aura of this field is infinite. Hence, the shortcomings, if any, in this edition will be substituted in the next edition.

Pankaj Gupta
Vijay Kumar Sharma
Sushma Sharma

Contents

1 The Bountiful Himalayas 1
1.1 People and Knowledge Systems 7
1.2 Concept of Healing in Epic Sagas 15
References 18

2 Health and Folk Medicine 21
2.1 Categorization of Traditional Healing Systems 24
2.2 Folk Medicine: The Lesser Known Traditions. 25
2.3 Research Studies on Healing Traditions of the Himalayan Region 29
References 33

3 Ethnic Food as Medicament 37
3.1 Culinary Traditions of the North-Western Himalayas. 39
References 58

4 Mystic Healers 61
4.1 Mediators Between Materialistic and Metaphysical Worlds 66
4.2 Sacred Healing by Buddhist Monks 73
4.3 Plants in Magico-Religious Rituals 75

5 Traditional Herbalists 83
5.1 Dependence of Indigenous Mountain Communities on Forests 84
5.2 Herb Collection and Processing. 86
5.3 Methods and Collection Time 86
5.4 Collection Strategies 88
5.5 Processing of Medicinal Plants 88
5.6 Cultivation of Medicinal Plants. 89
5.7 Traditional Methods Employed for Preparing Herbal Formulations. 91
5.7.1 *Kwath*: Infusions (Hot Teas). 91
5.7.2 *Kadha*: Decoctions (Boiled Teas) 91

5.7.3 *Rasa*: (Extracts, Alcohols, Local Wines) 92
5.7.4 *Lepa*: (Concoctions, creams for external applications) . . . 92
5.7.5 *Churan*: (Powder of dried herbs). 93
5.7.6 *Vatti*: (Tablet). 93
5.7.7 *Dhuni*: (Inhalers/Snuffs). 93
5.8 Dosage System 94
5.9 Administration of Medicine 94
5.10 Traditional Therapeutic Procedures 95
5.11 Pediatric Medicine. 97
5.12 Indigenous Dermatology and Cosmetology 97
5.12.1 Pimples or *Acne vulgaris* 98
5.12.2 Scalds, Boils and Burns 99
5.12.3 Wounds 99
5.12.4 Leucoderma 100
5.12.5 Skin Care Cosmetics 100
5.12.6 Traditional Face Packs and Cosmetics 100
5.13 Scalp Conditions 101
5.13.1 Dandruff or *Pityriasis Simplex Capillitii* 101
5.13.2 Hair Care Cosmetics 101
5.13.3 Oral Care. 102
5.13.4 Cosmetics for Hands and Feet 102
5.14 Snake and Insect Bite 103
5.15 Generalized Health Problems 103
5.16 Ear Nose and Throat Problems 104
5.17 Eye Care 104
5.18 Urinary Problems 105
5.19 Managing Diabetes 105
5.20 Traditional Orthopedic Practitioners. 106
5.21 Managing Gastrointestinal Disorders 110
5.22 Handling Respiratory Disorders. 112
5.23 World of Traditional Birth Attendants 112
5.23.1 Knowledge of Handling Gynaecological Problems and Birthing 114
5.24 *Amchis*: Traditional Healers of Kinnaur 116
References 119

6 Indigenous *Materia Medica* 121
6.1 Material Used by Folk Herbalists 122
6.1.1 Medicinal Plants 122
6.1.2 Animal/Animal parts 133
6.1.3 Minerals/Salts. 133

Epilogue 137

Appendix A: Dried Herbs 141

Appendix B: Medicinal Plants 143

Appendix C: Medicinal Plants 145

Bibliography 147

About the Book 149

Figures

Fig. 5.1 Buffalo horn used for blood letting. 109
Fig. 5.2 Blood letting expert depicting the procedure 109
Fig. 5.3 Amchi traditional medicine man. 117

Tables

Table 1.1 Plant genetic diversity of Himachal Himalayan 6
Table 3.1 Food consumption pattern during pregnancy 42
Table 3.2 Food consumption pattern of a lactating mother. 44
Table 3.3 List of foods restricted or prescribed for common body discomforts 45
Table 4.1 Plants used in Magico-religious Practices 78
Table 5.1 Geographical distribution of forest in Himachal Pradesh 85
Table 5.2 Powder and tablet(s) suggested for treating acne 99
Table 5.3 Plants used for the treatment of diabetes 106
Table 5.4 Formulation used for neuro-muscular disorders 108
Table 5.5 Plant species reported by traditional midwives and herbalists for managing infertility. 115
Table 5.6 Formulations reported by traditional midwives for managing gynaecological problems 115
Table 6.1 *Materia Medica* of traditional system of medicine (Appendices A–C) 124
Table 6.2 Therapeutic utilization of animal/animal parts 133
Table 6.3 Therapeutic utilization of minerals 134

About the Authors

Pankaj Gupta is Senior Research Officer at the Institute of Integrated Himalayan Studies (IIHS), University Grants Commission (UGC) Centre of Excellence, Himachal Pradesh University, Shimla, India. He is a doctorate in Biosciences from Himachal Pradesh University and the Managing Editor of *Himalayan Studies Journal* & IIHS News Bulletin. He is also a member of the editorial team of *Himshikhar*, the Himachal Pradesh University Newsletter, brought out quarterly by Himachal Pradesh University, Shimla. He is member of the Mountain Forum Himalayas, a non-government organization active in the Indian States of Himachal Pradesh and Uttarakhand, and has been an expert for project evaluations funded by the Council for Advancement of People's Action and Rural Technology (CAPART), India. He has been a consultant for the Himachal Pradesh Power Corporation Limited for social impact assessment studies and baseline studies since 2008. His areas of interest include village studies, natural resource management, health-oriented problems of women and children, traditional healthcare systems and magico-religious methods of healing, ethno-ecological, and audio-visual documentation of culture and nature.

Vijay Kumar Sharma is Project Officer at the Institute of Integrated Himalayan Studies, University Grants Commission (UGC) Centre of Excellence, Himachal Pradesh University, Shimla. He has published papers in reputed journals, besides editing and authoring two books. He has been involved in various research projects of the Institute funded by the UGC and other funding agencies. His areas of specialization are rural sociology, folk medicine, and indigenous knowledge.

Sushma Sharma is Professor in the Department of Biosciences, Himachal Pradesh University, Shimla. She was previously the Director of the Women's Study Centre of Himachal Pradesh University. She has completed a number of projects funded by the UGC and other funding agencies. Dr. Sharma has worked on nutritional and physiological studies of Himalayan people. Her research papers have been published in journals of national and international repute. Her area of specialization is muscle physiology.

Prologue

...The art of medicine is entertaining the patient
while Nature cures the disease....

Voltaire

With the dawn of the twenty-first century, man has realized the damage caused due to depleting bioresources and containment of folk traditions which is a matter of concern. In the globalized era, the local traditions are giving way to contemporary thinking. These changes are affecting occupation patterns, means, and earnings and socio-cultural milieu of indigenous societies. In this process, the understanding that local communities have developed over the years, is fading into oblivion.

Nevertheless, indigenous knowledge holds a key position in the lives of deprived sections of society. It is one of the main components of social capital of the unprivileged, their main asset to endow in the struggle for endurance, to raise crops, to provide a safe refuge to mountain communities, and to fight against ailments. Traditional wisdom that has evolved within the communities, and confined to specific cultures, forms the basis for decision making and survival strategies. It encompasses important issues linked with primary production, human and animal life, natural resource management, etc. (UNESCO, 2002).

The traditional wisdom, which is based on novelty, adaptation, experimentation, is orally transferred from one generation to another. "Traditional Knowledge" or "folk wisdom" is a testimony of accomplishments of human civilizations in realizing the intricacies of life and survival. This knowledge may be methodological, social, organizational, or cultural, attained as a part of great human experimentation intended for evolution and survival. The importance of safeguarding the traditional knowledge and its cultural and ecological resource base is crucial, mainly in the context of globalization and extensive demand for natural resources. It is valuable not only to those directly concerned with it, but also to contemporary psycho-social care, primary healthcare, preventive medicine, agriculture, animal husbandry, forestry, etc. For instance, traditional knowledge linked with forest management originates from man's relationship with nature and that relationship leads to more sustainable methods of farming and using forest products. Moreover, the time-tested wisdom can be used to elevate the contours of indigenous knowledge and its custodians. This not only has consequences for the continuance of long-established practices within the communities, but also for the linkages established outside communities. The traditional knowledge systems are open and informal and can be used for enhancing the conventional scientific knowledge which is closed and formal. Modern science is based on theories and principles, while the indigenous knowledge systems rely on values, beliefs, and customs. The long-established methods of natural resource management, for example, are not applicable to a particular community, but to the people of the outside world, living in identical conditions.

Folk knowledge is invaluable in many respects. It not only provides local expertise, but also bestows useful indications for future scientific development. Appropriate policy interventions, capacity building including responsive youth and documentation of indigenous knowledge systems can regenerate fading folk traditions. The local healthcare systems offer a wide range of variations including the folk health traditions and magico-religious healing. In Himalayan regions, many folk traditions are still playing an important role in the local healthcare sector. This monograph traces the origin, status, and prospects of local healing traditions in the North-Western Himalayas.

The traditional Himalayan Medicine System is an example of the traditional knowledge system where small communities living in fragile ecosystems fight against diseased states by making use of timeworn healing traditions. People not only rely on these conventional methods for their own existence, but also for their crops and livestock. Rural communities make use of traditional wisdom for handling diseases of domestic animals and also in farm management practices. These folk remedial measures are completely oral, non-documented, and make use of plant products such as latex, resin, bark, root, leaves, fruits, etc., minerals, animal products, and magico-religious practices.

The Himalayas has a rich legacy of folk medicine and other indigenous healthcare practices. Besides *Ayurveda*, a number of ethnic healthcare systems remained widespread in the Himalayas. The *Ayurvedic* system of medicine is a codified system, which was evolved more than 2000 years ago and is based on early classical Sanskrit treatises, while the ethnic healthcare practices were developed by the indigenous communities through trial and error method, making use of locally available material of vegetal and animal origin. The topographical variation in the entire North-Western Himalayan region has shaped the complex geographical diversity, meteorology, and floral and faunal wealth. The region is home to a number of communities who enjoy living in harmony with the rich and unique elements of biodiversity. As elsewhere in the world, ethnic communities in the Himalayan region to a greater extent rely on local resources for fulfilling their routine needs. At higher reaches, folk healing is the only accessible form of health care for a majority of the communities, both logistically and economically. Medicinal plants are the main constituents of folk medicines and are, thus, of great importance in traditional healthcare. In most cases, the medical preparations contain a number of ingredients varying in proportion and are prepared according to the condition of patients. However, the method of preparation of formulations is confined to specific communities because of a chance of its mishandling. The knowledge of healing is unique and is known only to a few elderly folk. These restorative measures make use of locally available medicinal plants and play a significant role in the healthcare sector of inaccessible mountainous regions.

Traditional methods of health care were passed on from one generation to another either through "Gurukula"[1] mode of instruction or word of mouth. In many cases, the knowledgebase was kept confined to a few families. The trainees used to live with the trainer and learnt the art of healing from their masters, who have tried to uphold the long-established oral traditions. They were trained to prepare the medicine, method of drug administration, together with general care of patients. Even today, one finds the repository of old manuscripts in the Himalayan region, which contain the information on medicinal plants, their uses, method of usage, and contraindications. These manuscripts are considered holy, and most of them were learnt by heart. It was only after exhaustive learning and practice that the learner could become a self-sufficient practitioner. The art and skills of healing were passed on to the learners completely, but at a pace determined by the trainers. The trainees were not supposed to visit any formal school or taught any predefined set of courses. Their claim to practice was dependent only on the information provided by the trainers. Thus, after years of training these trainees become expert healers and before trying any medicine on their patient, they familiarize themselves with the ailment and body composition of their patient.

Materia Medica is an inventory of raw drugs obtained from plants, animals, and minerals employed in traditional healthcare systems. It is a Latin term used for the body of knowledge dealing with the curative properties of any material used for therapeutic purpose. In Latin, the phrase actually means "medicinal material." The phrase has been in use from the days of the Roman Empire until the twentieth century, but nowadays it has been substituted by the term pharmacology. *Sushruta Samhita*, attributed to *Sushruta*, is the earliest *Ayurvedic* treatise on medicinal substances. It describes more than 700 herbs, 64 preparations from mineral sources, and 57 preparations based on animal sources. The Greek physician Pedanius Dioscorides, in the first century AD, used the term *materia medica* for his pioneering works on medical matter in five volumes. It is a precursor to all contemporary pharmacopoeias, and is believed to be one of the most significant herbal reference guides in history. The most primitive Chinese *materia medica*, the *Shennong Bencao Jing*, was gathered during the Han dynasty and was attributed to Shennong. In the medieval Islamic period, Muslim botanists and physicians extensively worked on the earlier knowledge of *materia medica*, for instance, *Al-Dinawari* described more than 600 plant drugs, *Ibn al-Awwam* described more than 500 microbiological cultures, and *Ibn al-Baitar* described more than 1,000 plants, foods, and drugs. The investigational scientific technique was introduced into the field of *materia medica* by Andalusian-Arab botanist Abu al-Abbas al-Nabati, the teacher of *Ibn al-Baitar*. He introduced empirical techniques in testing, description, and identification of numerous *materia medica*, and segregated unproven reports from those supported by authentic tests and observations. This facilitated the evolution of the science of pharmacology.

---

[1] *Gurukul* (*Guru* refers to "the teacher" or "the master"; *Kul* refers to the domain, meaning extended family) was a kind of residential school in India where the students used to live in proximity with the teachers, and learn different skills from them.

Avicenna's *The Canon of Medicine* was the first pharmacopoeia, which listed 800 tested drugs, plants and minerals, followed by pharmacopoeias written by Abu-Rayhan Biruni, and *Ibn al-Baitar*. The origin of clinical pharmacology dates back to the middle ages in Avicenna's *The Canon of Medicine*, Peter of Spain's *Commentary on Isaac*, and John of St Amand's *Commentary on the Antedotary of Nicholas*. Canon introduced clinical trials, randomized controlled trials, and efficiency tests. During the middle and thec modern eras, *Materia Medica* was transformed to modern systematic discipline of pharmacology.

The *Ayurvedic Materia-Medica* is a storehouse of medicinally valuable drugs, which can cure several non-curable diseases. Unlike conventional, synthetic and fractionally isolated drugs of contemporary medicine, which have side effects, *Ayurvedic* medicaments make use of natural products, and these are used in semi-processed form and as a result have numerous benefits in addition to curing a disease. However, the traditional healthcare systems, which used to be the lifeline of remote areas, are on the verge of extinction. The number of traditional birth-attendants, bone-setters, and other folk healers, whose services were utilized most, is slowly diminishing. The rich information on traditional methods of healing, which still exists in the form of unrecorded *materia medica* of tribal communities, is slowly losing ground, and the custom of passing this knowledge on to the next generation is declining.

Even today, in many areas, this knowledge is kept a secret. Another popular conviction among the healers is that making money from a secret can render the treatment ineffective. A further important cause for this deplorable state of affairs is the lack of knowledge and faith among youngsters on the occurrence, characteristics, curative properties, and methods of using plants for therapeutic purposes. This is the reason for discarding the conventional technologies among the younger generation. The excessive exploitation of herbal material by pharmaceutical companies has resulted in considerable depletion of plant resources. But the rate of erosion of traditional knowledge is even more rapid than the rate of erosion of resources. Given the non-availability of requisite raw materials in their exact quantity and quality at the right time may jeopardize traditional healing practices. In view of the limitations on the extraction of medicinal herbs, together with the impact of modernization, people have started using allopathic drugs and, as a result, traditional healers are losing their identity.

The present situation calls for a well-organized strategic plan to safeguard and promote traditional healthcare systems, involving people in cultivation, processing, and promotion of medicinal plants and related knowledge. In the following pages, effort has been made to share the information gathered from healers of the North-Western Himalayas, which will certainly help in bringing the invaluable knowledge into limelight and preserving the same.

Reference

UNESCO. (2002). Best Practices Using Indigenous Knowledge. Retrieved from 5 March, 2013 http://www.unesco.Org/most/Bpikpub2.pdf.

Chapter 1
The Bountiful Himalayas

> *...tongues in trees, books in the running brooks, Sermons in stones, and good in everything...*
>
> Shakespeare
> As You Like It

Abstract The indigenous wisdom and practices remained the basis of subsistence of traditional mountain communities. Rich in bio-resources and indigenous knowledge, the Himalayan region is truly a sacred land, where nature has conferred its unrivaled treasure to its inhabitants. From the times of yore, the mighty Himalayas have acted as the meeting ground for different races, cultures, religions, etc. and nurtured the world's greatest civilizations. Really, the Himalayas acted like a guardian and prevented its natives from various invasions. The entire range offers daring expedition to unearth the hidden treasures. North-Western Himalayas has varied climatic conditions which favor floral, faunal and cultural diversity. The region is a home of many indigenous and ethnic groups. Entire region has a rich legacy of folk medicine and other indigenous health care practices. There is a long tradition of using herbs both for preventive and therapeutic purpose by indigenous societies. Indian medical history is filled with galore of sage-cum-physicians who augmented the fields of science. Mountain communities have sufficient knowledge regarding identifying, harvesting, utilizing and preserving herbs in their natural habitats for sustainable utilization. The traditional knowledge is available in the form of oral narrations lacking scientific credentials, which needs to be documented, preserved and utilized for the betterment of mankind.

Keywords North-western Himalayas · Himachal · Genetic Diversity · Traditional knowledge · *Ayurvedic* medicine · Chinese medicine · *Unani* medicine · Traditional knowledge systems

For centuries, the snow-clad mountains and sacred rivers have nurtured the great civilizations of the world and are the meeting ground for different races, cultures and religions. With 2,400 km length and varying width of 240–330 km, the Himalayas, consist of three ranges-the greater Himalayas, the lesser Himalayas, and the outer Himalayas. In addition to this, there is a fourth, northernmost range,

P. Gupta et al., *Healing Traditions of the Northwestern Himalayas*,
SpringerBriefs in Environmental Science, DOI: 10.1007/978-81-322-1925-5_1,

known as the Trans-Himalayan range. The southern slopes of the Himalayas are enormously steep to support the vegetation, while the northern slopes, generally lie below the tree line and are covered with forests. Between these ranges are widespread plateaus, deep gorges, and fertile valleys. The Himalayas play a key role in shaping the climate of the entire region by offering a physical screen within which the monsoon system operates. From amidst the Himalayas, originate the great river systems which are the source of water for all alluvial plains. Further, the Himalayas are known for their historical, religious and geographical significance. Historically, the Himalayas acted like a protector and prevented its inhabitants from various invasions. The entire range offers daring expedition to unearth the hidden treasures. People throughout the world have travelled and are still taking a trip for enjoying its beauty. With the famous silk route, the region connects the Central and the South Asia, thus creating a bridge between the culturally and religiously diverse countries. The region has witnessed and catered to the oldest Indian Civilization. The twin cities of *Mohenjo-Daro* and *Harappa* were discovered in the foothills of the Himalayas. The early Aryans used to consider the Himalayas as the abode of Gods and Goddesses.

The evolution of the Himalayas dates back to millions of years ago. The Himalayas are among the youngest mountain ranges and consist mostly of uplifted sedimentary and metamorphic rocks. According to the plate tectonics theory, the Himalayas are formed as a result of continental collision between Indo-Australian Plate and Eurasian Plate. The tectonic movement between the two plates raised the deposits of shallow Tethys Sea and shaped the Himalayas. The Indian Himalayan Region holds an unusual status in the mountain ecosystems around the globe. The Himalayas, which separates the Indian Peninsula from the Central Asia, due to its diverse flora, fauna, geography, ecology, socio-cultural and aesthetic values has great sacred and environmental significance. The entire region is rich both in biological resources and traditional wisdom. Since earlier times the indigenous knowledge and practices have been providing the basis for the welfare and livelihood of mountain communities, maintaining their wellbeing and reinstating its environment. Rich and untouched natural resources, which are found in its vicinity, have not only taken care of numerous civilizations but are essential for the sustenance of generations to come. The region with its diverse altitude, environment, rainfall and soil conditions has greatly influenced the human resources. Having acted as a natural and political barrier for centuries, the Himalayas have cultivated and propagated a number of traditional knowledge systems, customs and communities, who in spite of living in unreachable valleys have endorsed their cultural individuality.

The Himalayas are personified as Himavath, the father of *Goddess Parvati*, and while describing its legacy, the famous Indian poet, Kalidas wrote that the Himalayas are imbedded with valuable stones; covered with countless herbs having immense worth. He called the Himalayas as amazing delight of Lord Shiva. The whole region is considered as the realm of Lord Shiva- the supreme ascetic,

'*Pashupati'*—the compassionate supreme of shepherds. Personified as awfully sacred, with height as an invariable tribute to the distinction of human soul and its immensity, the Himalayas exemplify universality of self-realization. The Himalayas have summoned sages, *yogis*,[1] artists, philosophers, researchers and writers from all over the world. Adi Shankaracharya, a famous Indian saint, established one of the four cardinal hermitages in the Garhwal hills. Swami Vivekananda laid the foundation of *Mayavati Ashram,* 50 km from Almora. Scientist J. C. Bose, ventured into the Himalayas to explore how the Ganges flows down from the 'matted locks of Lord Shiva'. The Mughal emperor, Jahangir, describing the beauty of the snow covered peaks of Kashmir, said, *'If there is a paradise on the earth, it's here'*. *Rig Veda*,[2] the ancient Hindu scripture, gave Himalaya, the status of a deity. *Sama Veda*[3] inscribes Himalaya as the center of globe. In *Mahabharata*,[4] one finds that Yudhishtra,[5] the eldest brother of *Pandavas*,[6] soared the Himalayan peaks seeking ecstasy, and the pursuit was named as *Swargarohan.*[7] *Skanda Purana*,[8] one of the sacred Hindu scriptures, propounds that one can be liberated from all transgressions by simply gazing at the Himalayas. Several tales are intertwined with the Himalayas and these mythologicals strengthen the belief system of people who hold a belief that even a glance of mighty the Himalayas washes away all sins and opens doors for liberation. A number of folk deities are worshipped in every Himalayan village, and thus, the whole hill province is named as '*Devbhumi*'—the sacred land of deities. As an abode of peace, there are many references on the Himalayas as the place where sages have meditated in the pursuit of tranquility and the majority of associated myths have a base in the idea of penance. It is said that meditating on the Himalayas brings liberation which manifests in the form of true knowledge dispelling the darkness of ignorance and facilitates in achieving a pious state. It is generally said, just as dew vanishes with the sunrise, all sins get washed away at the very sight of the glorious Himalayas.

> …He, who thinks of Himalaya, though he should not behold him, is greater than he who performs all worship in *Kashi*…

---

[1] *Yogi* is a practitioner of *Yoga* or ascetic practitioners involved in deep contemplation.

[2] *Rig Veda* is an ancient collection of *Vedic* hymns in Sanskrit praising Gods which are still recited as prayers, during religious occasions.

[3] *Sama Veda* is the ancient sacred scripture and second of the four *Vedas*.

[4] *Mahabharata* is one of the two major epics of primeval India, the other being the *Ramayana*. The epic is part of history, which besides its epic account of *Kurukshetra* War, contains much theoretical material, pertaining to the four 'goals of life'.

[5] *Yudhishtra* was the eldest son of King *Pandu* of *Indraprastha*. He was known as *Dharmaraja*, for his goodness.

[6] *Pandavas* were the five sons of King *Pandu*, their names being *Yudhisthira, Bhima, Arjuna, Nakula* and *Sahadeva*.

[7] *Swargarohan* is a journey of soul towards heaven after liberation from body.

[8] *Skanda Purana* is the prime Hindu *Mahapurana*, a genre of eighteen religious texts, whose text is dedicated mainly to the miraculous life of *Subramanya*, son of Lord *Shiva* and *Parvati*.

In Tibet, Himalaya is worshipped as the mother of earth and looked upon as the supreme source of inspiration and insistence. According to Tibetan mythology, *Bodhisattva* made an outlet through Himalaya and with this originated Tasangpo, the great river of Tibet. The Bhutanese mythology claims that Guru Rimpoche came to Bhutan riding on a flying tiger where he rescued the place from demons and spread Buddhism in the region. Whether it is in Hinduism, Islam, Buddhism or Jainism, the Himalayas have remained a cradle of mythology making it more fascinating and spiritual.

The economy of the Himalayan region as a whole is a bit pitiable with the low per capita income. Much of the region is characterized by a very low economic growth rate combined with a high rate of population growth, which contributes to stagnation in the already low level of per capita gross national product. Most of the inhabitants are dependent on subsistence agriculture and modern industrial expansion is still lacking. Though the patches of agricultural land have been carved out in the mountainous forested areas, but the main agricultural land is concentrated in the *Tarai* region and Mid-Himalayan valleys. Rice is the main crop in the east *Tarai* region, while corn is common in the rain-fed hillsides, other cereal crops being wheat, millet, barley and buckwheat. A variety of fruits are grown in different zones of Himalayas. Tea and potatoes are other major crops. Food processing units, vegetable oil industries, small sugar refineries and brewing are some of the major industries, common in the region. Since early 1950's, tourism has emerged as a major expanding business. However, the unplanned economic transition and population increase are posing threats to Himalayan ecology. In the recent years, deforestation and overgrazing has resulted in soil erosion and other environmental problems, while, the rapid population increase has accelerated pollution problem, which plead for critical scientific consideration.

The North-Western Himalayan region consisting of the states of Jammu & Kashmir, Himachal Pradesh and Uttarakhand, is comparatively arid thus, characterized by famine tolerant and chill resistant plants. The region shows a wide altitudinal disparity ranging from tropical to alpine vegetation. Nearly 80% of the communities inhabiting the region depend on farming and allied activities for their livelihood and consequently known to have the genetic resource wealth of crop plants, their wild relatives and other important plants possessing nutritive and therapeutic value. The rich inter-specific diversity exists for the genera like *Avena, Amaranthus, Chenopodium, Fagopyrum, Allium, Hordeum, Linum, Pyrus, Prunus, Rubus, Fragaria, Sorbus, rosa, Lilium, Vicia, Lepidium, Lathyrus, Cucumis, Solanum* and *Trichosanthes* contributing considerably for the sustenance and improvement of traditional Himalayan agro-ecosystems. Wild plant resources found in Himalayan regions have satisfied the requirements of indigenous communities, by making available, fuel-wood, wild-edibles, raw-stuff for crafts, and herbs for health care.

Around 18,440 species of plants are found in the Indian Himalayan region of which about 45 % are having medicinal properties. The number of medicinal species in Himalayas is approximately 7,500–10,000 which contribute significantly to the biodiversity of the region. The Himalayas having a huge wealth of medicinal plants and traditional knowledge play a key role in the health-care systems of mountain societies. It is estimated that 70–80% of rural population depends on traditional medicine for primary health-care, even though allopathic medicine is available in many parts (Farnsworth and Soejarto 1991; Sheng-ji 2001). Medicinal plants, being important source of rural earnings in the region, add considerably to the economic development of the communities, and also support modern industrial development both inside and outside the region.

Himachal, one of the fascinating regions in the North-Western Himalayas, has varied climatic conditions which favour floral, faunal and cultural diversity. The state is a home of numerous indigenous and ethnic groups. Situated in the heart of western Himalayas, Himachal is bordered by the state of Jammu & Kashmir and Uttar Pradesh. Located between 30°22′ and 30°12′ North Latitude and between 75°47′ and 79°4′ East Longitude, the state has altitudes ranging from 350–7000 m above the mean sea level. Physio-graphically, Himachal can be divided into three zones; outer Himalayas or the *Shivaliks*, inner or the Middle Himalayas and the Greater Himalayas or the Alpines. With the total area of 55,673 km^2, the state has twelve districts namely, Kangra, Hamirpur, Mandi, Bilaspur, Una, Chamba, Lahaul and Spiti, Sirmaur, Kinnaur, Kullu, Solan and Shimla. Out of 12 districts, Kinnaur, Lahaul and Spiti and Pangi and Bharmour sub-divisions of Chamba fall in tribal area. The climatic conditions of the region are ideal for the growth of wide range of plants and herbs which provide raw materials for pharmaceutical, food, flavouring and cosmetic industries. Nearly 90 % of the people live in villages and small towns and their livelihood depends on agriculture and horticulture, besides livestock rearing.

Himachal derives its name from the word '*Himalaya*', which literally means '*Land of snowy mountains*'. The people of Himachal are simple, diligent and truthful. Women work along with men at home and also in the field. Besides this, women perform certain out-door and domestic chores. Institution of village Gods holds a very prominent place in the life of people who worship village deities and are inclined towards nature worship. Festivity and joy are the integral part of their simple spiritual life. The entire state is famous for pilgrimages, rituals, ceremonies, legends, and folklore. The state is rich in water and land resources. The main natural water sources are rivers, lakes and streams. The pristine *Chandrabhaga*, *Ravi, Beas*, *Sutlej* and *Yamuna* rivers are perennial, fed by snow and rainfall, and are protected by a wide cover of natural vegetation. Besides rivers, *Renuka, Rewalsar, Khajjiar, Dal, Beas Kund, Dasaur, Brighu, Prashar, Mani Mahesh, Chander Tal, Suraj Tal, Kareri, Sreolsar, Gobind Sagar* and *Nako* are the major lakes. A number of small water springs and rivulets also contribute to the resource wealth of the state. The state's economy is developing in all aspects, from self-sufficient agriculture to the infrastructure development for industrial expansion, along with the horticulture, transport, forest and hydel resources. The agricultural sector contributes over 45 % to the net state domestic productivity and nearly the entire rural population of state depends directly on agriculture. The people in state make profit by raising cash crops and main food crops grown are wheat, maize, rice, barley, seed-potato, ginger, vegetables, vegetable seeds, mushrooms, hops, olives, figs, etc. Fruit

Table 1.1 Plant genetic diversity of Himachal himalayan

Name of plant	Area
Rice	Dhauladhar belt, Changer belt, outer Saraj, Chidgaon and Jagatsukh area
Maize	Rajgarh and Shilai in Sirmour, Salooni, adjoining areas of Chamba, Chadiahar, Changer areas
Wheat landraces	Karsog, Changer, Bilaspur, Mandi and Hamirpur
Barley	Nako in Kinnaur, Pangi, Spiti, Outer Saraj, Changer area
Amaranthus	Sarhan, Kupvi, chopal, Nichar, Poda, Dodra Kawar, Shiali, Bara Banghal, Gusain
Buckwheat	Sangla, Neshang, Ropa valley and Dodra Kawar
Millets	Upper Mahasu, Pangi and parts of mid Kinnaur
French bean	Bara Banghal, Bharmour, upper Kinnaur and Outer Saraj
Kulthi	Bhatiyat, Chowari of Chamba and adjoining parts of Kangra
Field peas	Spiti Valley
Cowpea	Bandla area of Bilaspur, Changer area of Hamirpur, Kangra and Mandi
Kala zeera	Sangla and Pangi Valley
Wild chickpea	Spiti Valley
Cucurbits	Salooni and Banzradu area of Chamba, Changer areas of Hamirpur, Kangra, Mandi and Kandi area of Una
Chilli	Haripur and Nauradhar area of Sirmour, Banjaar area in Mandi & Kullu, Salooni and Mahlan areas of Chamba
Apricot	Pangi, Leo and Ropa, Spillo, upper Shimla, Pin valley in Spiti
Wild pomegranate	Darlaghat, Narag areas of Solan, Bhambla, Rewalsar, Drung areas in Mandi and Basantpur in Shimla
Almond	Spillo, Leo and Ropa, upper Shimla, Pin Valley in Spiti
Walnut	Pangi and Holi in Chamba, outer Saraj in Kullu, upper Kinnaur
Sea-buckthorn	Lahaul and Spiti, Upper Kinnaur

Source NBPGR, Shimla

cultivation also provided economic boom to the farmers and state is identified as country's Apple state. There is a rich genetic diversity for the vegetable crops and the region also has an advantage of growing off-season vegetables. The Regional Station of National Bureau of Plant Genetic Resources, Shimla, has made sincere efforts to maintain the Agri-horticultural diversity in the region and identified the hotspots of important food crops in the region. (Table 1.1)

Forests are the vital land resources and the state is blessed with a huge area under green cover. According to the Forest Survey of India report (2003), legally defined forest areas constitute 66.52 % of the total area of state, though the actual area under tree cover is only 25.78 %. Forest types mainly consist of moist tropical, dry tropical, mountain sub-tropical, mountain temperate, sub-alpine and alpine scrub. The southern part of Himachal has both tropical and sub-tropical dry and moist broadleaf forests. The vegetation in sub-tropical forests consists of *Shorea robusta, Dalbergia sissoo, Pinus roxburghii;* pine whereas the temperate region consists of oaks, deodar, blue pine, fir and spruce. The state forests are rich in vascular flora, which forms the conspicuous vegetation cover. Out of total 45,000 species of plants found in the country as many as 3,295 species (7.32 %)

grow in the state. Himachal aptly showcases the medicinal plant richness and the diversity of zone spreads over its different agro-climatic zones with vegetation types stretching from an altitude of about 300 m along the Punjab plains to more than 6,000 m along the inner Himalayan range. The state harbours more than 3500 species of flowering plants, out of which about 800 species are estimated to be used for medicinal purposes within and outside state. An analysis of the habits of state's medicinal plants shows that majority of these are herbs (70 %), followed by shrubs (15 %), trees (10 %) and climbers (5 %). Medicinal plant diversity in the state can also be appreciated from the fact that its medicinal plants are spread across more than hundred plant families with the highest represented families being *Asteraceae*, *Rosaceae*, *Ranunculaceae* and *Fabaceae*. Knowledge about the medicinal plant diversity and conservational efforts has placed the state on the herbal map of the country drawing the nature lovers and entrepreneurs from far thereby boosting its economy.

Ecosystem specific use of plants for health care is a very strong living tradition of our country. The ancient scriptures and mythology are full of references on healing plants from the Himalayas. In Himachal, a number of plants are used for health care purpose, which are spread across different agro-climatic zones in the state and make a significant contribution towards the human and veterinary health security. The people of the state enjoy customary 'right' to collect medicinal plants from state forests and common lands in their vicinity for their household consumption. The depletion of these resources is affecting the traditional practices related to health care. This depletion could result in permanent loss of rich knowledge base associated with these herbs, which otherwise should be taken care off.

1.1 People and Knowledge Systems

Hinduism is probably the only religion which supported science and scientific discoveries. Origin of most of the contemporary inventions can be traced in ancient Hindu scriptures. According to ancient texts, around 3000 BC Sage Kapil founded both cosmology and psychology. His *Sankhya*[9] philosophy covered the secret levels of psyche, including mind, intellect and ego, and how they are related to the Soul or *Atma*. Around this era and through 400 BC, many great developments occurred. In the field of medicine, sage Divodasa Dhanwantari developed the school of surgery; *Rishi* Kashyap developed the specialized fields of paediatrics and gynaecology. SageAtreya,[10] author of *Charak Samhita*,[11] classified the

[9] *Sankhya* is one of the six orthodox schools of Hindu philosophy and classical Indian philosophy. Sage Kapila is traditionally known as the founder of this school.

[10] *Atreya* is a descendant of *Atri*, one of the great Hindu sages whose accomplishments are detailed in the *Puranas*.

[11] *Charak Samhita* or the "Compendium of sage *Charaka*" is an early text on Indian traditional medicine. It is one of the two foundational texts of this field.

principles of anatomy, physiology, pharmacology, embryology, blood circulation and discussed the mechanism of healing thousands of diseases, many of which modern science still has no answer. Along with herbs, diet and lifestyle, Atreya showed a correlation between mind, body, spirit and ethics. Sage Atreya has written about the causes and cures for diabetes, tuberculosis and heart diseases. At that point of time, the Europeans had no knowledge about diverse fields of science. While sage Atreya is recognized for his contribution to medicine, sage Sushrut is known as the "Father of Surgery" and author of *Sushrut Samhita.*[12] Modern science also recognizes India as the first country to develop and use rhinoplasty. Sushrut also practiced amputation, caesarean, cranial surgeries and developed more than hundred surgical instruments—many of them look similar to instruments used nowadays; and discussed more than 300 types of surgical operations. Sushrutha considered the head as the centre of all special senses, and described cranial nerves connected with specific sensory functions. Sushrut divided 1,120 diseases into natural and supernatural. He taught palpation and auscultation of heart, lungs and womb and advocated the use of special senses. He was the pioneer of most teaching techniques in experimental and clinical surgery.

Indian medical history is filled with galore of sage-cum-physicians who enriched the fields of science such as medicine, surgery, astrology, etc. Sage Nagarjuna wrote many famous books including *Rasratnakar*, which describes the methods of extraction and preparation of many metals like gold, silver, tin, copper, zinc, etc., and their uses in healing. His *Uttaratantra* deals with preparation of medicinal drugs. Nagarjuna introduced addition of metallic compounds into *Ayurvedic* drugs which was mainly dealing with herbs and vegetable products until then. Sage Agnivesa was one of the earliest writers of ancient Indian health and medicinal system called *Ayurveda.* He was disciple of sage Atreya Punarvasu. According to *Charaka Samhita*, Lord Indra taught *Ayurveda* to Sun God, who passed it on to sage Atreya Punarvasu, who in turn passed it on to six of his disciples namely Agnivesa, Bhela, Jatukarana, Parasara, Harita and Ksarapanii. Sage Charaka who wrote *Charaka Samhita*, a treatise on *Ayurveda*, was disciple of sage Agnivesa. *Charaka Samhita*, a masterly book on *Ayurveda* was written by his disciple sage *Charaka.*

Ancient treatise on medical systems and its development includes, *Agni Purana*,[13] which has mentioned treatment of cattle and horse, *Garuda Purana*[14] talks about the treatment of horse and elephants, *Shalihotra Samhita,* an ancient text, describe the treatment of diseases in horse. *Matasya Purana*[15] older treatise by

---

[12] *Sushrut Samhita* is a Sanskrit text on surgery, attributed to *Sushruta*, a historical physician of 6th century. It consists of 184 chapters, description of more than 1000 illnesses, 700 herbs and preparations from mineral sources and based on animal sources.

[13] *Agni Purana* is one of 18 *Puranas* and contains about fifteen and a half thousand verses.

[14] *Garuda Purana* is one of the *Puranas* which are part of the Hindu body of texts known as *Smriti*. It contains details of life, after death, funeral rites and the metaphysics of reincarnation.

[15] *Matasya Purana* is one of the oldest Post-Vedic Hindu scriptures called the *Puranas.* It narrates the story of *Matsya* (Fish), the first of ten incarnations of Lord *Vishnu*.

Pakapya muni and *Somaputra Budh* illustrates the treating techniques for diseased fishes. In *Shyama Shastra,* an ancient manuscript, one comes across the treatment of birds, especially pigeons. There are a number of accounts about the veterinary physicians in Hindu epics. Sage Dronacharya trained *Nakula* and *Sahdeva* in treatment of horses and Nakulais said to have authored a treatise on horses. One comes across a number of incidences which display the evolution of medical sciences in the ancient period. In *Rig-Veda,* one finds a reference of artificial limb and method of investigating ears. In *Mahabharata,* there is a mention of micro-organisms and chromosomes. *Aitereya Upanishad*[16] describes the development of embryo in the body and sixteen functions of brain. *Shrimad Bhagwat* explains the process involved in cell division and also explains that a disease producing agent is capable of preventing or curing the disease. In *Ramayana*, king Dasharatha asked queen *Kaikayi* to seek the advice of royal physicians for getting relief from her illness which clearly indicates that medical profession existed at that time. Once Sage Gautama castrated the testicles of Indra and *Ashwins* transplanted the testicles of goat and saved Indra. This indicates that physicians of that time were aware of organ transplantation. The knowledge of toxicology finds mention in numerous ancient scriptures. *Shrimad Bhagwat* is filled with references which reinforce that people were well aware of science of toxicology. In *Mahabharata*, various types of serpents have been described. The great epic poem holds that Lord Brahma passed on the knowledge of toxicology to Sage Kashyapa.

People knew the art of preserving a dead body. The dead body of the king Dasharatha was preserved in "*Taila Droni*"[17] till the arrival of Bharat. Death incidence of *Ravana* indicated that *Ravana* had died because of injury to his *Naabhimarma* due to arrow of Lord Rama. This is the reference of 107 sensitive points which were known at that time. In the enumeration of '*Madhushala'* of Ravana, different types of *Asavas*, wines, meat and their preparations according to the principles laid down in *Ayurveda*, several varieties of *sura,* or the wine and the vessels made up of gold, silver, quartz, etc. have been described, which shows that the science of fermentation and the use of alcoholic preparations was known to the ancient people.

Epic *Mahabharata* of *Vedavyasa* is one of the greatest epics of Indian literature. It highlights different aspects of *Ayurveda* including its eight branches and various types of medical and surgical treatments. Once sage Narada went to king *Yudhishthira* and made enquiry about his health, which shows that the practice of medicine already existed in those days. There is a mention of incidence of parthenogenesis and tube baby in *Mahabharata.* It holds that the embryo of the *Kauravas* emerged from the womb of Gandhari in the form of a single egg. But, when it did not grow into a baby for a long time, Gandhari beat herself on her abdomen which resulted in abortion. The pieces were kept separately, one in each earthen pot containing clarified butter for a period of ten months. As a result one

---

16 *Aitereya Upanishad* is one of the Upanishads commented upon by sages such as *Adi Shankara* and *Madhvacharya.*

17 *Taila Droni* is an ancient method of healing which make use of oils for treating diseases.

child engendered from each piece. *Mahabharata* also narrates an incidence where the zygotes formed in the uterus of Kadruva and Vinata were kept in earthen pots containing clarified butter gave birth to children.

In *Santiparva* section of epic *Mahabharata*, the episodes of psychosomatic disorders and their clinical signs have been described along with the influence of *Trigunas* on the body and mind. Many of the great saints and seers of ancient times were not born of the usual human birth, but appear to have been modified in some kind of cosmic test-tube or artificial birth. References are found in the ancient texts, for instance, sage Agastya and his brother, *Vasishtha*, were born from the seminal fluid of the Gods Mitra and Varuna which was placed in earthen pots. In Jain mythology, one finds that the soul of Lord *Mahavira* first got embodied as an embryo in the womb of a *Brahmin* mother, but later, the Gods transferred it into the womb of a queen. A similar transference of embryo of Balaram from the womb of Devaki to that of Rohini is described in the *Vedic* literature. Similar to these, there are numerous examples of resorting to ritualistic performances not only for healing but also for obtaining progeny of one's own choice.

The Himalayas host the three largest traditional medical systems of the world: *Ayurvedic* medicine, Chinese medicine, and *Unani*[18] medicine. The use of herbal medicine dates back as far as the Indus Valley civilization in 2600 BC. Chinese and *Ayurvedic* medicine developed by local people are used even today. This type of knowledge is very significant to contemporary pharmaceutical research as it acts like an initial screen which can help isolate the medically significant properties of plants and animals. Utilizing the traditional wisdom, numerous modern drugs, including anti-cancer drugs, antibiotics, malaria drugs, and analgesics, have been developed from animal and plant resources.

One finds countless instances in literature which illustrates the development and utilization of ancient healing techniques. There is a long tradition of using medicinal plants both for preventive and curative health-care by rural societies. Local people have reliable facts and efficient techniques to recognize, harvest, utilize and preserve herbs in their natural habitats for sustainable utilization. This knowledge is not only used for curing human ailments but also to cure ailments of domestic animals. These techniques are available in the form of oral narrations and have no scientific credentials. The ethnic communities make use of herbal products, minerals, animal products and *tantric* practices for saving life. According to an estimate of the World Health Organization (2008), approximately 80 % of the people in developing countries are dependent on traditional medicine for fulfilling their primary health care needs and a major part of these employ medicinal plants. Understanding the indigenous knowledge systems of mountain people in relation to biodiversity, resource management and cultural traditions is essential for the growth of Hindu-kush Himalayan region, which requires identification of changes in resource management, culture, decision-making and tenure systems.

[18] *Unani* refers to a tradition of Graeco-Arabic medicine, which is based on the teachings of Greek physician Hippocrates.

In ancient times, and even today, the traditional wisdom and practices remained the livelihood basis of indigenous mountain communities. In modern times, the two are utilized by food, pharmaceutical, and cosmetic industry. Rich in bio-resources and indigenous knowledge, the Himalayan region is truly a blessed land, where nature has bestowed its unsurpassed treasure to the communities. Human resources, i.e. population, settlement and economic patterns within Himalayas are significantly influenced by variation in topography and climate, which impose severe restrictions on living conditions, restrict movement and impair communication. Nearly forty million people inhabiting the inaccessible and remote valleys of Himalayan region have preserved their cultural identities. Generally, Hindus of Indian heritage are dominant in Sub-Himalayas and Mid-Himalayan valleys from eastern Kashmir to Nepal. In central Nepal, the Indian and Tibetan cultures have intermixed, producing a blend of Indio-Tibetan traits. The Eastern Himalayas in India and nearby areas of the Eastern Bhutan are inhabited by animistic people whose culture is comparable to those living in Northern Myanmar and Yunnan province in China.

Having acted as a natural and political barrier for centuries, the Himalayas have nurtured a number of communities, cultures and customs. The Hindu epics talk about *Kiratas*,[19] *Kinnars*,[20] *Khasas*[21] and *Darads*,[22] who were original inhabitants of the Himalayas. Since early times, there have been migrations into the Himalayas. Spiritual quest motivated a few to migrate there, and a small minority responded to the call of mountains to test their own endurance and determination. Besides this, pursuit of profit propelled some others to approach Himalayas. The inhabitants of Himalayan region include, Bhytiyas of Bhutan and *Sikkimese* from Sikkim consisting of three different groups—*Lepchas*, *Bhutiyas* and *Nepalese*; *Ladakhis* from Ladakh and *Himachalis* of Himachal. Majority of Himalayan communities have sustained themselves by choosing agriculture and animal husbandry. Ethnic spectra of central and western Himalaya differ conspicuously from that of north-eastern region. Racially, a majority of tribal communities, particularly those in north-eastern regions, exhibit '*mongoloid*' features as can be observed from the physical features. Evolution, migration and acculturation gave rise to a diversity of socio-cultural identities representing tribal-non-tribal continuum.

The age-old and time tested Traditional Knowledge Systems (TKS) have evolved in the mountainous regions and facilitated the survival of people in extreme climatic conditions. Until recently, it was traditional wisdom that provided a vast majority of people with the basis for production of daily needs, activities including, farming, irrigation, artisanal creation, healthcare, childcare, etc. Berkes (1993) defined traditional knowledge as:

---

[19] *Kiratas* are the ethnic people inhabiting the Himalayan region.

[20] *Kinnars* are the tribal people, inhabiting the tribal district Kinnaur having a well-organized political and administrative set up.

[21] *Khasas* are an Indo-Aryan ethnic people who inhabit district Kangra, Mandi, Kullu, Shimla, Sirmaur and Kinnaur of Himachal Pradesh, as well as of Kumaon-Garhwal.

[22] *Darads* are people belonging to ethnic Himalayan tribe.

> A cumulative body of knowledge and beliefs handed down through generations by cultural transmission, about the relationship of living beings (including humans) with one another and with their environment. Further, traditional knowledge is an attribute of societies with historical continuity in resource use practices; by and large, these are non-industrial or less technologically advanced societies, many of them indigenous or tribal

According to International Indigenous Forum on Biodiversity:

> Indigenous knowledge is the essence of the identities and world views of Indigenous peoples. Traditional knowledge constitutes the collective heritage and patrimony of Indigenous peoples. Therefore it is priceless to us, and its value cannot be calculated for economic exploitation.

Traditional knowledge has many definitions but the central theme consisted of cultural beliefs and traditions being passed on from forefathers to the present generation for the purpose of survival while communities still live in harmony with the ecosystems. Traditional knowledge is something that is learned during a lifetime and realizes the interconnectedness of trees, soil and water. Traditional knowledge is based on the experience and observation over the years, and is hidden in folklore, oral tradition, myths, legends, ceremonies and songs. Its validity is demonstrated by the survival of techniques that have been successfully used by countless generations and need no authentication of occidental sciences. The traditional knowledge distinguishes one society from another. For some communities, this knowledge has a personal and spiritual meaning, reflecting their interest while, many rely on it for their survival. Its relevance has been acknowledged by Global Science and suggested that scientific and traditional knowledge must be integrated in interdisciplinary projects.

Epics are full of instances which narrate the legacy of people and knowledge systems which have helped in the survival of civilizations. *Puranas*[23] enumerates 14 extraordinary types of *vidyas* or knowledge, thereby enunciating their usage and benefits to the humanity. *Anulepana*[24] *Vidya* explicates how with the use of a particular '*lepa*' or paste, an individual can walk miles together, without any physical pains. There is a reference of '*Sweccharupadharini*[25] *Vidya*' which can help a person change his appearance as per his wish. *Vedic* literature contains numerous tales where people, such as, king *Darmamurti*, demon *Mahishasura*,[26] and many others were skilled of changing their appearance as per their desire. *Astragamarhudya*[27] *Vidya* is related to the use of weapons for attaining victory

---

[23] *Puranas* are spiritual texts, including the narratives from creation to demolition, lineages of emperors, legendary heroes, theorists and accounts of Hindu cosmology and ideology.

[24] *Anulepana* is act of applying ointment, paste, cream or lotion on body.

[25] *Sweccharupadharini* is the art of assuming different forms at one's own desire.

[26] *Mahishasura* is the name of a demon, whose narratives are available in the Hindu mythology.

[27] *Astragamarhudya* is the knowledge which deals with the weapons and art of wining. According to Hindu mythology this knowledge was passed by a scholar, named *Manorama* to king *Manu*.

over enemies. *Sarvabhutaru*[28] *Vidya* enables a person to construe the language of animals, birds, insects, etc. *Pamini*[29] *Vidya* helps in revealing hidden treasures, whereas *Rakshoghna*[30] *Vidya* provides security from the ill-minded being, which is intended to upset the organization of holy rituals. *Jalandhari*[31] *Vidya,* teaching the tactics of battlefield, was passed by sage Valmiki to Lav and Kush. *Parabala*[32] *Vidya* helps in achieving spiritual powers. This knowledge helped *Arjuna* in viewing various forms of Lord *Krishna*. *Purushapramodini*[33] *Vidya* helps females to hypnotize men. *Ullapanavidhana*[34] *Vidya* is one of the wisdoms which help in healing body aliments particularly related to bones. This knowledge helps, in straightening the twisted things. Lord Krishna straightened the deformed body of *Kubja*[35] by making use of this knowledge. *Devahuti Vidya* could help summon the Gods. *Yuvakaran*[36] *Vidya* can revitalize anything. *Vajravahanika*[37] *Vidya* can helps spot and kills enemies in disguise. A man can acquire supernatural powers with the help of *Vajreshwari Vidya*.[38] On the other hand, *Gopalamantra Vidya*[39] provides a skill in speech to make things come true. In addition to these, the other lifesaving knowledge which developed over a period of time in ancient India, includes, *Mritsanjeevani vidya*[40] and *Karanpisachini vidya*.[41]

The people prescribing traditional medicines lack formal scientific knowledge about disease, but pursue their specialties, by learning through observation and

---

28 *Sarvabhutaru* is the knowledge which facilitates a person to construe the language of animals, birds, insects, etc. According to Hindu mythology, a scholar called *Vibhavari* blessed *Manu* with this wisdom.

29 *Pamini* is the wisdom which enables a person to find hidden treasures.

30 *Rakshoghna* is the knowledge by which the malicious upset the ritualistic performances.

31 *Jalandhari* is a wisdom, which according to Hindu mythology, was passed by sage *Valmiki* to *Lav* and *Kush*, two sons of Lord *Rama*.

32 *Parabala* is the skill of imparting spiritual powers and according to Hindu mythology, lady Tripura, bestowed this knowledge on *Arjuna*, which enabled him to view Lord Krishna's cosmic self.

33 *Purushapramodini* is the art of hypnotization and finds its mention in epics and holy treatise.

34 *Ullapanavidhana* is the art of straightening the twisted things. Lord *Krishna* used this knowledge to uncurl the deformed body of a lady known by the name *Kubja*.

35 *Kubja*, according to the great epic *Mahabharata*, is said to be one of the female servants of king *Kansa*, and was known to possess deformed body. It is after the blessings of Lord *Krishna*, that she was revived back to normal from her physical ailment.

36 *Yuvakaran* is the process by which any old object could be revived to young form. Legendary queen *Shakuntala* was known to possess this knowledge.

37 *Vajravahanika* is the art by which one could mark and destroy opponent in disguise.

38 *Vajreshwari* is the knowledge associated with vanquishing of enemies.

39 *Gopala mantra* is the knowledge by which one could attain ability in the speech to turn out things true.

40 *Mritsanjeevani,* written by learned *Sukracharya*, is a knowledge, which offers protection all kind of diseases.

41 *Karanpisachini vidya,* a process of achieving mystic powers which can equip a person to read the mind of others.

imitation. Often healing is passed on from one generation to another. The folk healers use combination of prayer, charms and rubbing or massage; or prescribe herbal teas or decoctions of herbs or animal parts. People not only use native herbal medicines for treatment of common ailments like cough, cold, fever, headache, body-aches, constipation, dysentery, burns, cuts, scalds, boils and ulcers, skin diseases, respiratory troubles, etc., but these systems have remedies even for many incurable diseases like cancer, leucoderma, snakebite, diabetes, rheumatism, asthma, etc. The herbal remedies are often prescribed by household ladies, elder persons, folk healers, like *Pujari*[42] or *Ojhas*[43] and traditional herbalists. Magico-religious therapies make use of various procedures as *Jagar*,[44] *Thau-dham*,[45] *Tantra-mantra*,[46] etc., to appease the local deities and supernatural powers.

The household condiments and spices are utilized by rural women for curing common health problems of infants and children. In addition, the use of infusions of *Ocimum sanctum* leaves for cough, cold and mild fever; *Curcuma domestica* for cuts, burns and scalds; *Piper nigrum* fruits for cough and cold; *Trachyspermum ammi* seeds for stomach troubles, etc., are few familiar household remedial measures. The village elders and priests are aware of herbal formulations, which are considered effective. These herbal formulations are recommended for common health disorders and normally, healing is done free of cost. Nature has bestowed its best for the mighty Himalayas, the land and water resources are plenty, but there is need of sustainable utilization of these. At the same time, the importance of safeguarding and management its resources and associated knowledge is very crucial, particularly in context of globalization and increasing demand of resources. This knowledge is not only important to those who are directly involved and linked with it, but also to the modern medicine. This not only has implications for continuation of traditional practices within communities, but also for interactions established outside the communities.

The Himalayan region, characterized by diverse biophysical environment, rich cultural milieu, has nurtured its ethnic groups and indigenous societies, since times immemorial. Because of its inaccessibility and poverty, the mountain systems remained neglected. The natural settings of Himalayas have also influenced resource management giving rise to numerous eco-zones, within which is found a large diversity of micro-climates and micro-environments. Biological resources are very varied; vegetation types are highly diverse and endemism is high. The Indigenous knowledge of Himalayan communities has played a very significant

---

[42] *Pujari* means priest.

[43] *Ojhas* are exorcists.

[44] *Jagar* is a Sanskrit word means to 'wake'. In this process—a spirit is invoked in the body of living human being.

[45] *Thau-dham* is a traditional Tibetan therapy.

[46] *Tantra-mantra* primarily deals with the spiritual practices and ritualistic worship, which aim at liberation from the cycle of birth and death.

role in the management of natural resources. However the developmental activities, overgrazing, expansion in agriculture land, etc., have resulted in depletion of natural resources and paving way for several problems such as land degradation, soil erosion, drought, etc., which require thoughtful consideration of scientific community.

1.2 Concept of Healing in Epic Sagas

The world is full of numerous anecdotes associated with the mythical healing Gods. The classical myth holds references of the most famous Asklepian[47] myth, which shows that Greeks and Romans expected the physicians to practice their art of healing irrespective of their social status. Asclepius is depicted as physician-hero in the first myth and then as a physician-God, the ideal physician to whom people in ancient Greece and Rome turned for healing and relief from physical and mental suffering. The cult of Asclepius was well-accepted during the 300 BC. These centres, known as an Asclepieion were used by priests to cure the sick. The process of healing was known as incubation, and the patient was made to spend a night in the dormitory. During the night they would apparently be visited by the God in a dream. Priests use to interpret their dreams and recommend a remedy, advice or remedial measures with a recommended visit to the baths and gymnasiums. Similar toAsclepios, Agwu is considered as the deity of health and divination in Lgbo mythology. While in *Maya* mythology, Ah Kin who is also the Sun God is prayed at sunrise and invoked to cure disease and to bring wives to unmarried men. In the Gallo-Roman religion, Alaunus or Alaunius is a Gaulish God of sun, healing and prophecy. Glanis was a Gaulish God associated with a healing spring located in the town of Glanum in the Alpilles Mountains of Province in Southern France. There are cisterns at the site of springs, where pilgrims bathe. Near one of them is alter to Glanis and the Glanicae was set up. The Glanicae were a triad of local Mother-Goddesses associated with the healing springs. In Roman mythology, Pilumnus was considered as a nature deity. He ensured the proper growth and health of children. Ancient Romans made an extra bed after the birth of a child in order to seek the help of Pilumnus. *Vejovis,* a Roman God was one of the first Gods to be born. He was a God of healing, and was later associated with the Greek Asclepius. In Roman mythology, Verminus is believed to protect cattle from disease.

In the religious system of Orisha worship, Babalu Aye is known as the spirit of illness and disease, who is associated with insanity, aging, illness, disease and death, and as the deity that cures the same. Basamum was the God of healing in pre-Islamic South Arabia. His name is believed to be derived from the proto-Arabic *basam*, or balsam, a plant that was used in ancient medicines. In Lusitanian

---

[47] *Asklepian* is the ancient Greek God of healing.

and Celtic Polytheism, *Borvo* was a healing deity associated with bubbling spring water. Similarly, Derzelas was a Thracian chthonic God of abundance, health and human spirit's vitality. Ebisu is the Japanese God of medicine and good health. In Etruscan mythology, Fufluns was a God of plant life, happiness, health and growth in all things. In classical Celtic polytheism, Grannus was a deity associated with spas, the sun, fires, healing thermal and mineral springs. He seems to have embodied the idea of therapeutic heat.

Han Xiang a Chinese God was believed to give life with his flute. Iron-Crutch Li, yet another Chinese God was benevolent to poor, sick and needy, whose pain and misery he alleviates with unique medicine from his gourd. Lu Dongbin is a historical figure and also a deity revered by many in Chinese cultural sphere, especially by Taoists for keeping healthy. Wong Tai Sin is a Chinese deity popular in Hong Kong having the power of healing. Zhongli Quan is a Chinese God who possesses a fan which has the magical ability of reviving the dead. In Aztec mythology, Ixtlilton was the God of medicine and healing, and therefore alluded to as the brother of Macuilxochitl, the God of well-being or good luck. *Kumugwe* in Pacific Northwest has the power to view the future, heal the sick and injured, and bestow powers on those whom he favours. Ningishzida is a Mesopotamian deity of medicine, and is considered as a God of nature and fertility. Mullo, a Celtic God, known from inscriptions is associated with Mars in the form of Mars Mullo. Pilgrims visit the shrines and present coins to the God, along with votive images of the afflicted parts of their bodies. Nodens is a Celtic deity associated with healing, sea, hunting and dogs.

Xu is arguably the main God of the Bushmen of South Africa. He is considered a benevolent and omnipotent supreme being. He is also considered as the sky God to whom the departed souls meet. He is said to "Summon the magicians to their profession, and bestow them with supernatural powers." He is thought to provide rain and is invoked in illness, before hunting and before travelling. Besides these, Agathodaemon, Apis or Hapis, Atepomarus, Belenus, Cunomaglus, Elder Zhang Guo, Dian Cécht, Erinle, Heka, Imhotep, Lan Caihe, Miach, Namtar, Shamash and Osiris are some other Gods associated with healing around the world.

Islam takes a holistic approach to health. When one part is injured or unhealthy, the other parts suffer. If a person is physically ill or injured it may be difficult to focus on anything but the pain. Speaking to his followers Prophet Muhammad spoke of the strong believer being better than a weak believer, in the eyes of God. The word strong here means strength in faith or in character, but it can equally mean health. Holy Quran is considered as a book of guidance, filled with mercy and healing. The holy Quran is not a treatise on medicine, but it does contain guidance that promotes good health and healing. Quran is a healing for the body and the soul. Whenever life becomes too tricky or one is beset by injury, illness or unhappiness *Quran* lights the way and lighten the burdens. It is a source of solace and ease. The words and verses of *Quran* contain a healing for humankind's woes and ills. It includes verses and chapters which could bring about healing from disease and distress. A number of similar miracles are mentioned in the New Testament of Bible which talks about the healing done by Jesus Christ. The Gospel of Mark narrates about a man named *Bartimaeus* being present and healed, as Jesus left Jericho. In the cleansing ten lepers' miracle, Luke states that while on his way to Jerusalem, Jesus sent ten lepers, who had sought his assistance, to the priests, and that they were healed. Healing the paralytic at Capernaum appears in Matthew. The synoptics state that a paralytic was brought to Jesus on a mat; Jesus told him to get up and walk, and the man did so.

The immense potential in the power of *Shabda* or the cosmic flow of sound hidden in music was recognized by great Indian sages and they devised several musical patterns emanating from the '*Omkara*' for chanting of the *Vedic* hymns for distinct spiritual effects. According to the *Vedic* philosophy, *yoga* and music both are part of *Nada Vidya*. *Yoga* deals with realization of the sublime sound of the eternal force of cosmic consciousness while music pertains to the perception and expression of the infinite spectrum of the rhythmic flow of the perceivable sonic currents pervading in nature. Both have direct impact on the seven wheels hidden along the spinal column and hence affect the physical as well as subtle bodies.

Indian mythology consists of a gamut of teachings and wisdom which includes the knowledge of *Ayurveda*. It is said that the formation of universe began with the will of Lord Brahma. His desire manifested when Purusha, i.e. cosmic consciousness and *Prakriti* i.e. nature and material energy came together. After this, Lord Brahma created *Ayurveda*, the science of life, for the benefit of mankind and passed its knowledge first to king DakshaPrajapati[48] and later to Ashwins,[49] the twin physicians of Gods and then to Lord *Indra,* the King of Gods. According to Hindu mythology, Lord Dhanvantari is considered as the God of *Ayurveda*. He is believed to be the incarnation of Lord Vishnu and finds mention in *Vedas* and *Puranas* as the physician of the Gods and one of world's first surgeons. Even today, he is prayed for seeking blessings for sound health. Lord Dhanvantari is depicted with four hands, holding medical herbs in one hand and a pot containing rejuvenating divine nectar called *amrita* in another. The *Puranas* state that Lord Dhanavantari emerged from the 'Ocean of milk' and appeared with the pot of divine nectar during the churning process of ocean by Gods and demons. *Vraddha Sushrutha* contains 120 chapters focusing on *Sutra Sthana* (fundamental principles), *Nidana* (etiology), *Sarira Sthana* (anatomy and physiology), *Cikitsa Sthana* (therapeutics) and *Kalpa Sthana* (toxicology). Other chapters are on training and attributes of a surgeon, surgical instruments and dreams. In the *Sutra Sthana,* four different types of diseases are described which include *Agantuka* (traumatic or extraneous origin), *Sarira* (bodily), *Manasa* (mental) and *Swabavika* (natural).

Thus, spirituality and religion have always been indispensable components of health and well-being. In contemporary times, the role of religion in medicine encompasses practices such as the use of meditation and prayer, pastoral

---

48 *Daksha Prajapati* was a legendry king who was born out of the right thumb of *Lord Brahma* and all people are believed to be his descendants.

49 *Ashwins,* in Hindu mythology are divine twin sons of *Saranya*, a Goddess of clouds and wife of Sun. The *Ashwins* are *Vedic* Gods symbolizes sunrise and sunset. They are the doctors of Gods and *Ayurvedic* medicine.

counselling, evoking forgiveness and compassion, engaging the mystery of death in end of life care; and looking for new dimensions in illness for patients and families as well as the health professionals who work with them. Integrative medicine recognizes and promotes the value of linking spirituality with the healing process. In the past several decades, it has become widely accepted that religious belief and practices have a significant impact on both physical and emotional health. Contemporary medical and scientific research has demonstrated that religious commitment aids in the prevention and treatment of emotional disorders, disease and enhances recovery. Thus, belief in and submission to the will of God is the most important part of good health care. It is believed and time-tested that recitation of God's divine name can cure hearts and minds, as well as overcome illness and injury. In this mechanical world, life is full of stress and strains which often disturb human beings. Everybody desires peace, prosperity and healthy life. There are various options such as allopathic medicine, homeopathy, *Ayurvedic*, holisticpathy, yoga, naturopathy, etc., to help individuals. On this critical juncture, the concept of healing propounded by epic sagas is one of the ancient and natural sciences followed in India and in rest of the world million years ago but lost glory in transition. This age-old miraculous knowledge should now be geared up with better understanding for the better health and life of future generations. One has to understand the need of the hour which is indicating to peep into the past and learn the essentialities of heath and healing systems.

References

Berkes, F. (1993). Traditional ecological knowledge in perspective. In J. T. Inglis (Ed.) *Traditional ecological knowledge: Concepts and cases*. Ottawa: International Program on Traditional Ecological Knowledge and International Development Research Centre.

Doles, J. (2003). *Healing scriptures and prayers*. Seffner: Walking Barefoot Ministries.

Farnsworth, N. R. & Soejarto, D. D. (1991).Global importance of medicinal plants. In O. Akerele, V. Heywood, H. Synge (Eds.), *The conservation of medicinal plants*, pp. 25–51. Cambridge: Cambridge University Press.

Government of India (2003). Report Forest Survey of India (FSI).

Himalayas Retrieved March, 2013 from http://en.wikipedia.org/wiki/Himalayas

International Indigenous Forum on Biodiversity. (2003). Opening Statement – December 8, 2003, Item 7 Sub-Working Group II on Development of Elements of a Sui Generis System for the Protection of Traditional Knowledge, Innovations and Practices of Indigenous and Local Communities (UNEP/CBD/WG8J/3/7)).

Jain, M. C. (2005). Occult power of gems. The Astrology Center of America, 207 Victory Lane, Bel Air, MD.

Jakobsen, M. D. (1999). *Shamanism: Traditional and contemporary approaches to the mastery of spirits and healing*. New York: Berghahn Books.

James, R. (1989). *The faith healers*. Amherst New York: Prometheus Books.

Johari, H. (1996). *Healing power of gemstones in tantra*. The Astrology Center of America, Victory Lane, Bel Air, MD: Ayurveda & Astrology.

Joshi, G. C., Tewari, K. C., & Pandey, G. (1992). A review of indigenous system of medicine with special reference to herbal drugs. *Aryavaidyan, 3*(3), 173–179.

Kalakoti, B. S., & Pangety, Y. P. S. (1988). Ethno-medicine of Bhotiya tribe of Kumaun Himalaya. *Bulletin of the Medical Ethnobotany Research, 9*, 11–20.

Kapoor, G. S. (2007). *Gems & astrology, a guide to health, happiness & prosperity*. The Astrology Center of America, Victory Lane, Bel Air, MD.

Kapur, S. N. (1998). Prachin Bharat Mein Vigyan aur Shilpa. Retrieved March, 2013 from http://www.slidefinder.net/4/49china_20country_20paper/49chinacountrypaper/25096812

Kelvin, S. (2011). How you can heal the sick—the secrets to divine healing. Kindle Edition.

Mishra, P. L. (1985). Medicinal plants of Himalaya. *Himalayan Journal of Science, 4 & 5*, 65–80.

Narayana, A. (1995). Medical science in ancient Indian culture with special reference to Atharvaveda. *Bulletin of the Indian Institute of History of Medicine Hyderabad, 25*(1–2), 100–110.

Oli, K. P., & Dhakhal, T. D. (2008). *Traditional knowledge in Himalayan region*. Kathmandu, Nepal: ICIMOD.

Pathak, B. (2005). *Book of gemstones (gems in their occult & remedial powers)*. Victory Lane, Bel Air, MD: Astrology Center of America.

Pingle, A. (2003). *Indian music*. Udaipur: Sri Satguru Publications.

Prakash, U. (1978). Shushruta of ancient India. *Surgery, Gynecology & Obstetrics, 146*, 263.

Purohit, A. N. (1997). Himalayan medicinal plants-focus on Uttarakhand. In Gyanodaya Prakashan (Ed.), *Himalayan biodiversity: Action plan*. Nainital, India.

Raghunathan, K. & Dube, S. D. (1992).Dravyaguna (Pharmacology). In P. V. Sharma (Ed.), *History of medicine in India*. New Delhi: Indian National Science Academy.

Rajagopalachari, C. (1957). *Ramayana*. New Delhi: Bharatiya Vidya Bhavan.

Rajagopalachari, C. (1958). *Mahabharata*. New Delhi: Bharatiya Vidya Bhavan.

Raju, V. K. (1994). Antiquity of Indian medicine: Excerpts from Charaka Club.

Raju, V. K. (2003). Susruta of ancient India. *Indian Journal of Ophthalmology, 51*, 119–122.

Saklani & Mihan, P. (1998). Traditional practice and knowledge of wild plants among the ethnic communities of Garhwal Himalaya. *Puratattva, 29*: 89–99.

Selberg, T. (1995). Faith healing and miracles: Narratives about folk medicine. *Journal of Folklore Research, 32*(1), 35.

Shah, N. C., & Joshi, M. C. (1971). An ethno-botanical study of Kumaun region of India. *Economic Botany, 25*(4), 414–422.

Sharda, V. (2009). *Puran prabhavit himachali lok jivan*. New Delhi: Satyam Publishing House.

Sharma, P. J. (1931). Hindu medicine and its antiquity. *Annals of Medicine History, 3*, 318.

Sharma, P. V., & Sharma, A. V. (1992). Pharmacy in ancient India. In P. V. Sharma (Ed.), *History of medicine in India*. New Delhi: Indian National Science Academy.

Sheng-Ji, Pei. (2001). Ethno-botanical approaches of traditional medicine studies: Some experiences from Asia. *Pharmaceutical Biology, 39*(1), 74–79.

Sheshadri, T. R. (2003). *The curative powers of Holy Gita*. New Delhi: Hind Pocket Books.

Singh, B., & Saradananda, S. (2008). Ethics and surgical training in ancient india—a cue for current practice. *South African Medical Journal, 98*(3), 218–221.

Somvanshi, R. (1993). Prachin Bharat main Pashu Palan evum Pashu Chikitsha Vigyan (Hindi), Part I, Rajbhasha Anubhag. Izatnagar, Uttar Pradesh. India: Indian Veterinary Research Institute.

Somvanshi, R. (2006). Veterinary medicine and animal keeping in ancient India. *Asian Agri-History, 10*(2), 133–146.

Subbaarayappa, B. V. (1989). Indian astronomy: A historical perspective. In S. K. Biswas (Ed.), *Cosmic perspectives*. Cambridge: Cambridge University Press.

Tipton, C. M. (2008). Susruta of India, an unrecognized contributor to the history of exercise physiology. *Journal of Applied Physiology, 104*(6), 1553–1556.

Tripathi, V. N. (2008). Astrology in India. In H. Selin (Ed.), *Encyclopedia of the history of science, technology and medicine in non-western cultures*. Berlin: Springer.

WHO (2008). Traditional Medicine Strategy. World Health Organization, Geneva

Chapter 2
Health and Folk Medicine

...Healing is a matter of time, but it is sometimes also a matter of opportunity...

Hippocrates

Abstract The effort to realize and uphold an optimum state of health has always drilled the minds of men and as a result, a number of healing systems have evolved around the world. Communities have devised systems to alleviate the tiresome condition arising out of illnesses using their own technique, which vary from one community to another. Each culture has set outlook regarding the disease causation and these are rooted in their belief systems. There are several theories which not only explain the cause of disease but also community's health care seeking approach. Archaeological and existing genetic facts state that human population voyaged to the Indian subcontinent and their familiarity with herbs and other naturally accessible material is as old as human civilization.Folk medicine includes healing practices and ideas on health care which are limited to a particular group in a culture, and are generally transmitted orally or word of mouth. In India, folk medicine is highly conditioned by the impact of folk deities and, sometimes it is so deep rooted that medicine and folk deities become an integrated whole. Across the whole Himalayan Region, folk healers have a remarkable knowledge of herbs, accumulated through generations and they have been developing the health care traditions through constant experimentation and years of experience which is rooted in understanding and realistic considerations.

Keywords Folk medicine · Health · Ayurveda · Unani medicine · Traditional healing systems · Local health tradition · Traditional Chinese medicine · Indigenous health care traditions · Atharvaveda · Hakims · Vaidyas

The endeavour to achieve and maintain an optimum state of health has always exercised the minds of men since ancient times. As a result, a number of healing systems evolved across the globe. People have devised systems to mitigate the wearisome situations arising out of diseases using their own method, which vary from one community to another. Health, or poor health condition, was once only attributed to biological or natural conditions. Socio-biologists have confirmed that

P. Gupta et al., *Healing Traditions of the Northwestern Himalayas*,
SpringerBriefs in Environmental Science, DOI: 10.1007/978-81-322-1925-5_2,

the spread of diseases is greatly influenced by the socioeconomic status of individuals, ethnical traditions or beliefs, besides other cultural factors. From the times of yore, people in different parts of world have been trying to explore the causes of aliments and have engaged themselves in discovering remedial measures. Human societies around the world have evolved a well-defined pharmacopoeia and therapeutic procedures, be it is religious, secular or logical. Such therapeutic procedures are influenced by traditional knowledge and practices, customs and habits, charms and invocations, as well as constant process of trial and error backed by years of experience. Tribal concept of disease and treatment, life and death is as varied as their culture. Traditional system of medicine has evolved as a result of time-tested experience of people who have been eagerly monitoring the behaviour-pattern of animals and plants through the ages. And most of the time, folk medicine is based on remedies found in nature. In tribal communities, magic has also played a great role in the emergence of system of medicine. Folk medicine has a deep rooted background and its patrons are drawn from ancient communities. Thus, folk medicine is said to have a long and honourable history; much longer than present-day western medicine, whose roots go into hoary antiquity.

Every culture has set attitudes regarding the causation of disease which are rooted in their belief systems i.e., naturalistic, *Ayurvedic*, biomedical, etc. Constant changes in economy, therapy, technology and insurance influences the way communities view and respond to medical care. The sociology of wellbeing and infirmity takes into account the interface between society and health. At the same time, it also looks at health and illness in context of social institutions such as the family, work, school and religion. Social scientists look at how social life governs morbidity and mortality rates and vice versa. There are apparent differences in patterns of health and illness across societies. Patterns of global change in health care systems make it very important than ever to investigate and understand the sociology of health and illness. Community's health care perceptions have a deep bearing on the choice of medical care. It can slow down the precautionary actions, hinder or obscure medical care. The range of insight which the communities have on illness is significant—it varies from witchcraft to germs and poor immunity. According to Western thought, the body is considered as a complex machine which must be kept "geared-up" and sickness is taken to be the breakdown of machine. This differs with Eastern thinking in which health is considered as a state of balance between the physical, social and super-natural environment.

There are numerous theories around the world which not only explain the cause of disease but also community's health care seeking approach. According to Personalistic system of belief, illness is caused by the intrusion of a human being or a supernatural, possessing special power. If someone happens to disobey a social norm or a religious taboo, he or she may call upon the wrath of a deity which manifest in form of sickness or taken as divine punishment. Similarly, illness in many cultures is seen as penalty for not carrying out rituals linked with the adoration of ancestors. In many cultures, illness is accepted as the result of bad karmic action. Illness arising from personalistic causes can be treated through ritualistic performance, which is done by special practitioners. In the naturalistic system of belief, health is closely linked with the natural environment. A proper balance needs to be maintained for the same and when the balance gets disturbed, it resulted in illness. Biomedicine is based on the "body-as-machine" metaphor. This thought formed the basis of western medical practice. The health beliefs around the world are governed by permutation of these theories, and underlie the use of many conventional medicines and therapeutic practices.

Archaeological and contemporary genetic facts state that human populations migrated to the Indian subcontinent and their acquaintance with herbs and other naturally available curative matter and their use is as old as human civilization. The therapeutic wisdom that has evolved over the years is the outcome of trial and error and exchange of information among communities. The process of exchange and integration still continues, and the scientific community and public is becoming conscious regarding the value of folk medicine, which has brought *Ayurveda*, *Unani* and *Siddha* into the mainstream. The challenge nowadays is to combine the best of different healing traditions to meet the healthcare requirements of modern society.

Archaeological explorations carried out at different sites imply that therapeutic intercessions such as dentistry and trepanation were carried out as early as 7000 BCE in the Indian subcontinent. The importance that people of the Indus Valley civilization gave to herbs and the stress on cleanliness suggest a highly developed health management system. Trade routes linked the civilizations to other parts of the world and it is probable that botanical and medicinal commodities together with the knowledge were among the valued things of barter. The hymns of the Vedic period provide insights into diseases and their remedial measures. Most ailments, both physical and mental, were attributed to malicious spirits and treatments consisted of ritualistic performances, charms and incantations, medicines and surgical procedures. During the post *Vedic* period, when diverse cultures intermingled, there was growing understanding on health and well-being and many movements supported the free spirit of query, particularly in the field of medicine. The Buddhist and *Jaina* texts written in *Pali*[1] have enumerated the use of medicines, surgical trials, etc. essential for the health and well-being. The spirit of scientific enquiry influenced the intellectual world and in such a cultural milieu there emerged the formal scientific culture of healing, i.e. *Ayurveda*. Later, as a result of trade and exchange of herbs and knowledge, there was amalgamation of ideas and the *Ayurvedic* texts were translated into other languages. *Unani, Rasashastra,*[2] *Siddha*, and *Sowa-Rigpa*[3] were the other formal systems of medicine that were practiced in the subcontinent. *Unani* system of medicine originated in

[1] *Pali* is a literary language belonging to Prakrit language family and was initially written down in Sri Lanka during the 1st century BCE.

[2] *Rasashastra* literally means the "Science of Mercury".

[3] *Sowa-Rigpa* is traditional art of healing common in Tibetan communities.

Arabian countries incorporated the elements of *Ayurveda, Rasashastra, Yoga*[4] and *Tantra*.[5] However, even before the codification of medical knowledge into treatise, there was rich treasure of medical expertise in the subcontinent.

Classical *Ayurveda* has been augmented over the years through such communications and exchange with folk practices. Tribal Healing traditions of tribal people who had traditionally relied on forests for healthcare have made valuable contributions to the *materia medica* of conventional medicine. From 8th century onwards, texts called *Nighantus*[6] dealing exclusively with the *materia medica* of *Ayurveda* were composed. During the pre-colonial period, early Portuguese and Dutch settlers relied on the blooming healthcare systems they noticed in India. In the early period of the British East India Company, Indian health care knowledge and "native healers" were main resources for colonial organization. Later, after the settling of East India Company, many physicians assumed scholarly roles and Western medicine was looked upon as the leading system of medicine. After Independence, the government made efforts to recognize *Ayurveda*, *Siddha* and *Unani* at par with contemporary allopathic biomedicine. However, in the recent years, there has been increasing awareness in alternate therapies. Biomedical and *Ayurvedic* scientists are making attempts to integrate the two so as to have a holistic view of nature of disease in terms of modern biomedical notion (Perinchery 2013).

2.1 Categorization of Traditional Healing Systems

In India, folk medicine is highly conditioned by the impact of folk deities and, sometimes it is so deep rooted that medicine and folk deities become an integrated whole. *Ayurveda* has evolved as the natural way of healing or naturopathy and for centuries, it was the only system of medicine in the country. At the same time, the concept of *'Yin Yang'*[7] developed in China. With the passage of time, these systems progressed into independent branches of learning. These age-old systems, based on herbs and diet, offer an effective and mild ways of restoring health, with the minimal risk or side effects. Naturopathy based on an ancient and traditional system takes human beings back to the fundamental of nature. Natural cures cleanse the body and enhance the body's system to treat itself and protect itself from germs.

Local health tradition is a vague term mostly used to set apart ancient and culture bound health care practices, which existed before the evolution of modern scientific medicine. Some frequently used synonyms for local health tradition are

[4] *Yoga* is a generally known generic term for physical, mental, and spiritual disciplines which got evolved in ancient India.

[5] *Tantra* is a style of religious ritual and meditation that originated in medieval India.

[6] *Nighantu* is ancient pharmacology book written between the 12th and 14th centuries.

[7] *Yin Yang* represents the ancient Chinese perceptions of how things work.

indigenous, un-orthodox, alternative, folk, ethno, fringe and unofficial medicine or healing (Unnikrishnan 2004). While discussing the legal aspects, Stephan (1983) interpreted the term 'traditional medicine' in a broad sense as:

a. Formalized traditional systems of medicine such as *Ayurveda*, *Unani*, and traditional Chinese medicine.
b. The traditional healers as defined by an African expert group in 1976 is:

> A person who is recognized by the community in which he lives as competent to provide health care by using vegetable, animal and mineral substances and certain other methods based on the social, cultural, and religious background as well as on the knowledge attitudes, and beliefs that are prevalent in the community regarding physical, mental and social well-being and the causation of disease and disability.

c. The practice of chiropractic, naturopathy, osteopathy, homoeopathy and even Christian Science.

The definition of Jan Stephan encompasses all aspects of health care systems other than the modern medicine. However, Bannerman et al. (1983) uses terms such as ethno, folk, alternative, etc., as synonyms at micro level; in other contexts they denote different schools of health care practices. *Ayurveda*, *Siddha*, and *Unani* are the three major streams of Indian health care traditions whereas *Amchi,*[8] *Ayurveda* and folk medicine are the three major systems of health care in the state of Himachal which make use of natural products as raw drugs. *Ayurveda* is a scientifically codified and theoretically structured area of knowledge. The folk medicine, on the other hand, is a set of practices passed on from one generation to the next, most of which are oral. However, in the North-Western Himalayas all the streams are unified and function as synchronized systems. The inheritance of traditional health care system in the region is a result of the synthesis of all systems.

2.2 Folk Medicine: The Lesser Known Traditions

Folk medicine incorporates healing practices and ideas on health care which are confined to a particular group in a culture, and are usually transmitted orally or word of mouth. It may also be known as Traditional, Alternative, Indigenous or Complementary medicine. These terms are often comparable however, only Indigenous and Traditional medicine are well harmonizing with folk medicine, while others can be considered in contemporary context. History of folk medicine can be traced back as early as primeval Egypt in 3000 BC, despite the fact that much of contemporary medicine originated in Greece. The Greek manuscripts were afterward translated to Arabic and then undergone further investigations in the Islamic world. *Ayurvedic, Unani*, Traditional Chinese Medicine and medical

---

[8] *Amchi* is the traditional Tibetan doctor.

herbalism have inherited a rich legacy from folk medicine. It integrates crude medicinal herbs, syrups, decoctions and infusions and is practiced by a few vendors, *Hakims*[9] and *Vaidyas*[10] in the inaccessible areas. People in a number of developing countries, still relies on folk practitioners, including traditional birth attendants, herbalists and bonesetters who make use of locally available herbs to meet their primary health care requirements. A few folk preparations are of incredibly high therapeutic value.

Traditional medicine has maintained its reputation in a number of Asian countries, such as China, India, Japan and Pakistan. In the last few years, there has also been a growing interest in traditional and alternative systems of medicine in many developed countries. Medicinal herbs are the oldest known health-care products and their value is increasing, though its percentage varies depending on the ethnological, medicinal and historical background of a nation. The history of the relationship between plants and healing medications takes us back to the evolution of medicine itself. Evidences from ancient scriptures-the *Atharvaveda*[11] from India, the Petrie collection from *Kahun* in Egypt, and the *Avesta* from Persia demonstrates that early medicine was not only based on religion and supernatural world but also narrates the use of herbal, animal and mineral products. Traditional Chinese Medicine (TCM) has been using many conventional practices and most of the information on early Chinese medicine has been gleaned from the Yellow Emperor's Nei Ching. Artemisinin, a potent anti-malarial drug was derived from *Artemisiaannua*, a plant used in China for the treatment of malaria. TCM is linked to Chinese Cosmology as a system of beliefs based on the principles of *Yin* and *Yang*. *Yin* and *Yang* are connected via a circular harmony, which connotes well-being, good weather conditions and luck, while disharmony leads to sickness, catastrophe and bad luck. Chinese medicine tries to restore harmony by making use of acupuncture, herbs and food to recuperate and maintain health. Herbal medicine is a vital part of Traditional Chinese Medicine. Herbs are recommended to the patient by taking into account individual's health status. It is believed that the herbal formulations normalize the natural balance of the body. These may be in form of pills, powders, decoctions and raw herbs administered orally or as balms for external use. *Kampo*, a Japanese system of herbal medicine, has a long history, which precisely makes use of herbs to treat diseases. The distinct aspect of *Kampo* is its method of diagnosis, which is done through abdominal palpation. The system is based on the assumption that disease occurs as a result of a cacophony in the flow of Qi (energy).

Similarly, Traditional Vietnamese Medicine (TMV) lays emphasis on nourishment of blood and vital energy, rather than focusing on precise indications. The system of medicine is based on the effect of energy on the body. This energy is

---

[9] *Hakims* is the traditional *Unani* physician.

[10] *Vaidyas* is the folk herbalist.

[11] *Atharvaveda* is a sacred text of Hinduism and is one of the four Vedas, often called the 'fourth Veda'.

believed to be inherited from parents and extracted from food. The main methods employed by TVM are herbal medicine, acupuncture and moxibustion. Acupuncture is yet another traditional technique, where the acupuncturists insert tiny needles into precise points linked with the energy channels of the body, which encourages healing and free flow of energy in the body. Acupuncture treats many conditions including musculoskeletal disorders, headaches, respiratory disorders, gynecological problems, gastrointestinal disorders, as well as mental stress. Moxibustion, a traditional therapy makes use of *moxa*, or *mugwort* herb, which is converted to fluff after a series of processes and later burnt. This fluff is used together with acupuncture needles, or sometimes burn on a patient's skin.

Gua Sha or coin rubbing on the other hand is done to scrape away fever. It is one of the ancient techniques used to scrape away disease through sandy-looking objects. Cupping fire, or merely cupping, is a type of conventional art of healing found in number of cultures. It involves placing of glass, plastic, or bamboo cups on the skin. In traditional Chinese medicine, cupping is a system of applying acupressure by generating a vacuum in patient's skin. The therapy is used in the treatment of respiratory diseases and musculoskeletal disorders. Chiropractic healing evolved in the end of 19th Century by Daniel David Palmer, a magnetic psychotherapist from Iowa, USA. The tradition is based on connection between spine and nervous system and self-healing properties of human body. Homeopathy on the other hand, was initially pointed out by Hippocrates, but it was a German physician, Hahnemann, who established its basic doctrine. At present, Homeopathy has been incorporated in the National Health Care Systems of numerous countries.

The Indian System of Medicine has always recognized the medicinal value of plants, for instance the curative properties of *Rauwolfia serpentina* root in treating mental aliments was known at least 2500 years before the western countries recognized its therapeutic value in treating mental disorders. In early forties, Indian scientists isolated the active substances from *rauwolfia* and explored its value for treating high blood pressure. Resent clinical research has highlighted the role of *Bacopamonniera* as 'brain tonic'. In ancient system of medicine, the herb was widely prescribed by folk healers for treating memory-loss and finds its mention in old texts as *Medhyarasayana*. *Vinca rosea*, with its pink or white flowers popularly known as *Sadabahar*, or 'ever bloom' has been used in the contemporary medicine for treating Leukemia. Traditionally, the plant was used for the treatment of *diabetes mellitus*.

Folk medicine has been promoted by various folk communities. Unlike *Ayurveda*, this stream of health has no codified speculative foundations. Customs or traditional rituals rooted in the beliefs of communities formed its basis. Thus, folk medicine is a folk epistemology that brings together the diversity hidden in folklore. However, folk medicine can further be categorized as tribal or rural medicine. Many folk therapies are practiced by Indian tribes and rural people for curing diseases. For instance, oil massage therapy, which traces its roots back to 3000 years, can cure a variety of physical and mental diseases, strains and tensions, arthritis, spondylitis, paralysis, obesity, sinusitis, migraine and rheumatism; magnetic therapy, involves the use of positive forces of a magnet to treat diseases; mud therapy, which is regarded as 1000 years old therapy, involves the use of mud paste on body to protect against diseases such as migraine, insomnia, mental disorders, sinusitis, asthma, indigestion, arthritis, viral infection, general ill health, etc. A range of traditional therapies have been described for incurable diseases including *talam*[12] for treating insomnia, improving eyesight, curing skin disorders and headache; *Chakra Basti,*[13] for curing dyspepsia and alleviating constipation; *Greeva Basti*[14] for curing the cervical spondylosis and chronic pain in the neck region and *Netra Dhara*[15] for treating cataract and improving eyesight.

In addition, there are numerous folk traditions linked with curing of snake and insect bite, birthing, bone setting, curing of jaundice, herpes, etc. which are carried out by specialized healers. Apart from herbal drugs, communities have been making use of animal products in various medical preparations. Healing by using products obtained from animals is known as zoo-therapy. Zoo-therapeutic procedures have been developed by rural communities who live in close contact with natural world. The animal body parts are not only used for healing purpose but also in magico-religious purpose, both by aboriginal and western societies across the globe. In India, almost 15–20 % of *Ayurvedic* preparations are derived from animals and different ethnic groups use animal-derived substances for healing human ailments (Oudhia 1995).

Thus, though various developmental processes have led to the homogenization of cultures, contemporary societies are fighting against diseases and sufferings using their traditional therapeutic procedures. Traditional and complementary or alternative medicine provides an important health care service to persons both with and without geographic or financial access to allopathic medicine. It has confirmed efficacy in areas such as mental health, disease prevention, treatment of non-communicable diseases and enhancement of quality of life for people with chronic diseases as well as for the ageing population. The World Health Organization has encouraged and supported its member states in incorporating traditional and complementary or alternative medicine in national health care systems so as to ensure its genuine use.

---

[12] *Talam* is the process of applying medicated paste on the forehead of the patient.

[13] *Chakra Basti* is the process in which the *Bastior* the pot is applied to body's chakras, for instance, umbilical region.

[14] *Greeva Basti,* in Sanskrit the word *Greeva* refers to neck and *Basti* stands for a pot. So the process, in which lukewarm medicated oil is allowed to stand on back of neck, is called as the *Greeva Basti*. The process is very useful in maintaining normal structure and working of neck region.

[15] *Netra Dhara* is a special cleansing method of pouring herbal decoctions in eyes.

2.3 Research Studies on Healing Traditions of the Himalayan Region

Across the entire Himalayan Region, folk healers have a remarkable knowledge of herbs, gathered through generations and passed on through years of apprenticeship. The traditional healers in the region have been developing the health care traditions through constant experimentation and years of experience which is rooted in understanding and realistic considerations. Traditional wisdom of Himalayan communities is passed through proverbs, folklores, legends, customs and myths. These sources reveal how troubles emerge in life and how resolved by the combined efforts of a community. In the long history of local influences, there are deformations, distraction and alteration in folk healing practices on the negative side, and creativeness, revisions and improvements on the positive side. But, the folk systems have remained responsive to local needs and expectations.

Indigenous Health Care Traditions in the Himalayan region have two treatment methods- natural and supernatural. The natural method is indicative whereas the supernatural stream is etiological. The symptomatic way involves identification of disease by examining the symptoms followed by management using natural medicine. The super-natural methods allocate precise causes to diseases. However, the cause or etiology is considered different from modern medicine. According to the folk beliefs, the cause could be anything like wrath of deity, evil spirits or sorcery, black eye, violation of taboos, etc. In order to deracinate the cause of disease certain ritualistic performances are done. In the Central Himalayan region, a magical therapy, called *jagar* is practiced against diseases. According to people, this is the greatest cure for many non-curable diseases, especially the psychiatric disorders. *Jagar* is generally organized at night and takes one night or twenty-two nights depending upon the severity of the wrath of the local God.

People classify diseases into two categories (a) related to the body (b) related to mind and mystical world. The bodily ailments are cured by making use of herbal medicines, coupled with animal parts and psychosomatic diseases by using magico-religious practices coupled with herbal medicines. Healers believe that the efficacy of medicine is lost, if its formulation is exposed to strangers. Himalayan people consider that diseases are caused by discontentment of local deities and hence treat them accordingly. For treating such diseases, priests or mystic-healers play a significant role. The mystic-healers explain to people the cause of disease and provide remedial advice. If the cause is any spell of an evil-spirit, the healer treats the patient with the help of hymns and supposedly drives away the spirit. Such magico-religious ceremonies can be seen in any Himalayan village, even among the educated classes. *Thau-dam*, a traditional Himalayan therapy is practiced in the rural Himalayan region for liver troubles, stomach troubles, backache, etc. This therapy was also practiced by the ancient people and finds mention in *Ayurveda* as *agnikarma*. *Thau* therapy is normally practiced by the elder people of village and is obligatory for 6 months to one-year old children. In Tibet, the healing is done by *Sowa Rigpa*, meaning 'the science of healing'. The basic theory is to provide stability to the chief energies of the body. The practitioner makes use of antique apparatus to find the root cause of disease. Treatment is carried out by adjusting diet together with herbal medicines. The healing is based on Buddhist principles and close relationship between mind and body. Gurmet (2004) gave an account of *Sowa-Rigpa,* commonly known as Tibetan or *Amchi* medicine practiced in Himalayan regions throughout Central Asia.

Numerous studies have been carried out to document the folk healing practices of Himalayan region. Pant and Pandey (1995) studied the ethno-botanical wisdom of *Tharu* community living in Nainital district of Kumaon region. During the survey, enumeration of 179 plants was done out of which 42 were of value in *Ayurveda* system of medicine. Samal et al. (2004) made an effort to document indigenous health care systems and its significance in physical well-being of people inhabiting Central Himalayan region. Panday (2004) gave an account of time-tested remedy, popular among the aborigines of Gonda, Bahraich and Balrampur districts using seed fume of *Solanum surattense* against tooth and gum disorders. Garbyal et al., carried out study in Darma valley of Dharchula Himalayas which is situated in Kumaon region of Uttaranchal state and reported the rare herbs and shrubs like *Aconitum heterophyllum, Bergenia ciliata, Cordyceps sinensis, Dactylorhiza hatagirea, Hippophae tibetana, Picrorhiza kurroa, Swertia ciliata, Taraxacum,* etc. Hamayun (2006) studied the ethno-botanical wisdom of people of District Buner regarding the use of shrubs and trees. He enumerated ninety four different plant species used for different purposes. Bhatt and Negi (2006) evaluated the plants used for Medicare by the tribal people of the Jaunsar area of Garhwal Himalayas. Kunwar et al. (2006) examined the ethno-botany and traditional use of plants extracted from the vulnerable Alpine zone in Nepal. The results indicated that a large number of plant species are used as traditional medicines. Kunwar and Bussmann (2008) reported the indigenous knowledge of communities living in Nepal Himalayas. The study reported that nearly 55 % of the flora had medicinal value. Dhyani et al. (2010) generated the database on Ethno-botanical aspects of *Hippophae salicifolia* D. Don. which has immense multipurpose properties and is traditionally utilized for food, medicine, veterinary, fuel, fencing, agricultural tools and dye mordant. Tiwari et al. (2010) carried out study in the Nanda Devi Biosphere Reserve, Uttarakhand and documented the ethno-botanical uses of plants belonging to 40 genera and 26 families.

Pant and Samant (2010) undertook a trip in the Mornaula Reserve Forest of Kumaun, West Himalaya and evaluated the uses of plants in medicine and religious ceremonies. Phondani et al. (2010) conducted a study on the medicinal plants and knowledge of diseases among *Bhotiya* tribal communities in the *Niti* valley of *Alaknanda* catchment in Central Himalaya. Indigenous knowledge of local traditional healers was assessed and eighty-six plant species were identified which are used for the treatment of 37 common ailments. Kunwar et al. (2010) evaluated the traditional herbal medicine in far-west Nepal which has flourished in rural areas. Rokaya et al. (2010) documented the use of plants in traditional herbal medicine for treatment of human and veterinary ailments in Western Nepal. The team documented 161 plant species used for treating seventy three human and seven veterinary ailments.

Srivastava et al. (1984) intensively explored the Gurez valley, Kashmir from ethno-botanical point of view. During the exploration 258 species of the plants were collected, out of which 105, species were used in Indian system of Medicine. Sand and Badola (1987) carried out an ethno-botanical study of Jammu and Kashmir, which occupies the top most position in North-western Himalayas. Communities living in the area were depending upon local medicinal plants for cure of various ailments. Khan et al. (2004) recorded ethno-medicinal value of twenty seven plant species belonging to twenty families from Uri, Kashmir Himalaya. Khan et al. (2004) recorded the ethno-medicinal value of twenty-seven plant species belonging to twenty families from Kashmir Himalaya. Kumar et al. (2009) made an attempt to explore the knowledge of the native of Kishtwar, Jammu and Kashmir for curing diseases. The team documented seventy one ethno-medicinally useful plants grown in the region. An ethno-botanical survey was carried out by Shah et al. (2012) in Tehsil Budhal of District Rajouri to gather information from tribal communities on the ethno-medicines uses of plants.

Gupta et al. (1980) extensively explored district Ladakh from ethno-botanical and phyto-chemical point of view. During the exploration, more than 800 plant species were collected from different forest ranges and included about 250 medicinal plants used by the tribals, local inhabitants and folk healers. Gupta et al. (1981) carried out ethno-botanical and phyto-chemical screening of seventy High Altitude Plants gathered from Ladakh. Padam et al. (2000) studied twenty-two medicinal plants from Sapi Valley of Kargil district, Ladakh Himalayas, which are traditionally used for the treatment of various ailments in *Amchi* system of medicine.

The Sikkim Himalayas were explored by Srivastava and Kapahi (1991) and about 400 plant species of medicinal and aromatic values were found to be useful. Maiti et al. (2003) gathered information on medicinal uses of fifteen types of tubers, rhizomes or roots used by *Lepchas*, *Nepalese* and *Bhutias* medicine for different diseases and health care. Dolui et al. (2004) documented traditional methods of treatment among rural societies of Meghalaya. Maity et al. (2004) gathered information on medicinal uses of fifteen types of tubers, rhizomes or roots used for different diseases and health care by the inhabitants of North Sikkim. Acharyya and Sharma (2004) studied 35 medicinal plant species, from 35 genera belonging to 30 families in Assam. Folklore medicinal uses of 33 plant species belonging to 22 families used for various ailments among tribes of North Cachar Hills, Assam, were reported by Tamuli and Saikia (2004). Das et al. (2005) and his associates collected information on the use of *Jatropha curcus* for the treatment of dysmenorrhoea by the Koch-Rajbongshi tribe in Nalbari district of Assam. Ethno-botanical studies carried out by Khumbongmayum et al. (2005) in four sacred groves of Manipur revealed therapeutic applications of 120 plant species for the treatment of common ailments like skin disorders, ulcer, rheumatism, bronchitis, etc. Bhardwaj and Gakhar (2005) carried out ethno-botanical studies in the state of

Mizoram and documented the usage of wild plants by the native people for cure of cuts, wounds and blood-clotting properties of plants.

Jamir and Lal (2005) reported the traditional method of treating ailments using different vertebrates and invertebrates and/or their products by *Naga* tribes. Kala (2005) investigated medicinal plants used by the *Apatani* tribe of Arunachal Pradesh and documented 158 medicinal plant species used by them. In 2005, Kalita and his associates studied the plant and animal based folk medicine used by people of Dibrugarh district for treatment of ascites, body pain, carbuncle, diabetes, epilepsy, gastritis, obesity, piles, pimples and urinary tract infection. Medicinal value of herbaceous plants used by ethnic groups of North-Kamrup district of Assam was collected by Das et al. (2006). In a study carried out by Borah et al. (2006) in Dibrugarh district of Upper Assam, revealed the use of 38 plant species represented by 36 genera and 29 families for the treatment of various gastrointestinal diseases. In an ethno-botanical field survey carried out by Majumdar et al. (2006) documentation of medicinal use of 33 species of flowering plants used for the treatment of various ailments in the tribal areas of Tripura was done. An ethno-botanical study was carried out by Das and Tag (2006) in Arunachal Pradesh during which the use of medicinal plants was documented for the treatment of malaria, fever, bone fracture, anemia, snakebite, cancer, reproductive health, rabies, tuberculosis, diabetes and jaundice. Sajem and Gosai (2006) documented the traditional knowledge of medicinal plants used by the indigenous *Jaintia* tribes residing in few isolated pockets of northeast India. Nimachow et al. (2011) studied the ethno-medicines of *Aka* tribe residing in Arunachal Pradesh which play crucial role in the health care services of tribal society. Chakravorty et al. (2011) prepared a consolidated list of edible and therapeutic insects used in Arunachal Pradesh by two tribal societies. At least eighty one species of local insects were used as food among members of these two indigenous societies. Wangchuk et al. (2011) carried out ethno-botanical authentication and identification of Khrog-sman of Bhutan and identified the botanical names of 113 ‘Lower Elevation Medicinal Plants’ described in the Bhutanese traditional medical texts.

Chauhan and Chauhan (1988) carried out ethno-botanical surveys in Trans-Giri Area of *Sirmour* District of Himachal Pradesh and documented use of wild medicinal and aromatic plants growing in the area. Srivastava et al. (1991) reported 41 plants together with their uses from Lahaul and Spiti, Himachal Pradesh. Meenakshi and Chauhan (2005) reported plant species with their ethno-botanical uses in Shilli Wildlife Sanctuary of Himachal Pradesh. Kanwar et al. (2006) carried out research in six villages of *Kangra* district of Himachal Pradesh to study the application of plants at household level for treating various kinds of ailments. Sharma et al. (2006) collected data on traditional phyto-therapeutic applications used by inhabitants of Spiti valley, a cold desert in western Himalayas. Rawat and Kharwal (2011) reported the use of 22 medicinal plants by traditional healers of district Mandi in curing gynaecological problems. Gautam et al. (2011) reported the diversity of plant resources of Bilaspur district of Himachal Pradesh for their medicinal, traditional and edible uses. About 10 types of diseases related to stomach, mouth, cough, cold, skin, blood, vitality and strength, bones, muscles, and other like memory, swelling etc., were found to be cured by using the plant based medicines. The studies carried out by different researchers not only bring into limelight various techniques and methods opted by people for getting rid of disease, but also focus on their traditional wisdom and skills.

Thus, the sustenance of indigenous system of medicine depends on the accessibility of resources and is practiced among all Himalayan communities for curing various types of health disorders. However, different communities have distinct ethno-medico-religious practices which continue even though contemporary Medicare is available to them. Hence it would be wise to grow this arena of knowledge widely so as to develop a new horizon in the medical field.

References

Acharyya, B. K., & Sharma, H. K. (2004). Folklore medicinal plants of Mahmora area, Sivasagar district, Assam. *Indian Journal of Traditional Knowledge, 3*(4), 373–382.

Bannerman, R. H. O., Burton, J., & Ch'en, W. C. (1983). *Traditional medicine and health care coverage: A Reader for health administrators and practitioners*. Geneva: World Health Organization.

Bhardwaj, S., & Gakhar, S. K. (2005). Ethno-medicinal plants used by the tribals of Mizoram to cure cuts and wounds. *Indian Journal of Traditional Knowledge, 4*(1), 75–80.

Bhatt, V. P., & Negi, G. C. S. (2006). Ethno-medicinal plant resources of Jaunsari tribe of Garhwal Himalaya, Uttaranchal. *Indian Journal of Traditional Knowledge, 5*(3), 331–335.

Borah, P. K., Gogoi, P., Phukan, A. C., & Mahanta, J. (2006). Traditional medicine in the treatment of gastrointestinal diseases in upper Assam. *Indian Journal of Traditional Knowledge, 5*(4), 510–512.

Chakravorty, J., Ghosh, S., Meyer-Rochow V.B. (2011). Practices of entomophagy and entomotherapy by members of the Nyishi and Galo tribes, two ethnic groups of the state of Arunachal Pradesh (North-East India). *Journal of Ethnobiology and Ethnomedicine*

Chauhan, M., & Chauhan, N. S. (2005). Ethnobotanical studies in shilli wildlife sanctuary, Himachal Pradesh. *Ecology, Environment and Conservation, 11*(3/4), 395–398.

Chauhan, V., & Chauhan, N. S. (1988). Ethno-botany of Trans-Giri Area of Sirmour district of Himachal Pradesh. *Bulletin Medico Ethno Botanical Research, 3 and 4*, 106–122.

Das, A. K., & Tag, H. (2006). Ethno-medicinal Studies of the Khamti tribe of Arunachal Pradesh. *Indian Journal of Traditional Knowledge, 5*(3), 317–322.

Das, N. J., Devi, K., & Goswami, S. R. (2005). Report on the treatment of dysmenorrhoea by the tribes of Nalbari district, Assam. *Indian Journal of Traditional Knowledge, 4*(1), 72–74.

Das, N. J., Saikia, S. P., Sarkar, S., & Devi, K. (2006). Medicinal plants of North-Kamrup district of Assam used in primary healthcare system. *Indian Journal of Traditional Knowledge, 5*(4), 489–493.

Dhyani, D., Maikhuri, R. K., Misra, S., & Rao, K. S. (2010). Endorsing the declining indigenous ethnobotanical knowledge system of seabuckthorn in Central Himalaya, India. *Journal of Ethnopharmacology, 127*, 329–334.

Dolui, A. K., Sharma, H. K., Marein, T. B., & Lalhriatpuii, T. C. (2004). Folk herbal remedies from Meghalaya. *Indian Journal of Traditional Knowledge, 3*(4), 358–364.

Gautam, A. K., Bhatia, M. K., & Bhadauria, R. (2011). Diversity and usage custom of plants of South Western Himachal Pradesh, India—Part I. *Journal of Phytology and Ethnobotany, 3*(2), 24–36.

Gupta, O. P., Srivastava, T. N., Gupta, S. C., & Badola, D. P. (1980). An ethno-botanical and phyto-chemical screening of high altitude plants of Ladakh Part—I. *Bulletin Medico Ethno Botanical Research, 3*, 301–317.

Gupta, O. P., Srivastava, T. N., Gupta, S. C., & Badola, D. P. (1981). Ethno-botanical and phyto-chemical screening of high altitude plants of ladakh-II. *Bulletin Medico Ethno Botanical Research, 2*(1), 67–88.

Gurmet, P. (2004). Sowa-Rigpa: Himalayan art of healing. *Indian Journal of Traditional Medicine, 3*(2), 212–218.

Hamayun, M. (2006). Ethno-botanical studies of some useful shrubs and trees of district Buner, NWFP, Pakistan. *Indian Journal of Traditional Knowledge, 5*(3), 407–412.

Jamir, N. S., & Lal, P. (2005). Ethnozoological Practices among Naga Tribes. *Indian Journal of Traditional Knowledge, 4*(1), 100–104.

Stephan, J. (1983). A profile of traditional practices in the W.H.O. regions. In R. H. Bannerman et.al. (Eds.), *Traditional medicine and healthcare coverage*. Geneva: World Health Organisation.

Kala, C. P. (2005). Ethno-medicinal botany of the Apatani in the Eastern Himalayan region of India. *Journal of Ethnobiology and Ethnomedicine, 1,* 11. Retrieved February 2013, from doi:10.1186/1746-4269-1-11

Kanwar, P., Sharma, N., & Rekha, A. (2006). Medicinal plants use in traditional healthcare systems prevalent in Western Himalayas. *Indian Journal of Traditional Knowledge, 5*(3), 300–309.

Khan, Z. S., Khuroo, A. A., & Dar, G. H. (2004). Ethno-botanical survey of Uri, Kashmir Himalaya. *Indian Journal of Traditional Knowledge, 3*(4), 351–357.

Khumbongmayum, A. D., Khan, M. L., & Tripathi, R. S. (2005). Ethno-medicinal plants in the sacred groves of Manipur. *Indian Journal of Traditional Knowledge, 4*(1), 21–32.

Kumar, M., Paul, Y., & Anand, V. K. (2009). An Ethno-botanical study of medicinal plants used by the locals in Kishtwar, Jammu and Kashmir. *Ethnobotanical Leaflets, 13*, 1240–1256.

Kunwar, R.M. & Bussmann, R. W. (2008). Ethnobotany in Nepal Himalaya. *Journal of Ethnobiology and Ethnomedicine*, 4, 24. doi:10.1186/1746-4269-4-24

Kunwar, R. M., Kunwar, R. M., Nepal, B. K., Kshhetri, H. B., Rai, S. K., & Bussmann, R. W. (2006). Ethno-medicine in Himalaya: A case study from Dolpa, Humla, Jumla and Mustang districts of Nepal. *Journal of Ethnobiology and Ethnomedicine, 2*, 27.

Kunwar, R. M., Shrestha, K. P., & Bussmann, R. W. (2010). Traditional herbal medicine in far-West Nepal: A pharmacological appraisal. *Journal of Ethnobiology and Ethnomedicine, 6*, 35.

Maiti, D. C., Chauhan, A. S. & Maiti, G. (2003). Ethnobotanical notes on some unexploited plants used by Lepchas and Nepalese Communities of North Sikkim. In V. Singh & A. P. Jain (Eds.) *Ethno-botany and medicinal plants of India and Nepal* (Vol. 1). Jodhpur, India: Scientific Publishers.

Maity, D., Pradhan, N., & Chauhan, A. S. (2004). Folk uses of some medicinal plants from North Sikkim. *Indian Journal of Traditional Knowledge, 3*(1), 66–71.

Majumdar, K., Saha, R., Datta, B. K., & Bhakta, T. (2006). Medicinal plants prescribed by different tribal and non-tribal medicine men of Tripura state. *Indian Journal of Traditional Knowledge, 5*(4), 559–562.

Narnag, S. & Mitra, M. (1998). Indigenous knowledge and the treatment of disease in Abujhmarh. In *Contemporary studies in human ecology*. New Delhi, India: Kamla-Raj Enterprises.

Nimachow, G., Joshi, R. C., & Dai, O. (2011). Role of indigenous knowledge system in conservation of forest resources-a case study of Aka tribes of Arunachal Pradesh. *Indian Journal of Traditional Knowledge, 10*(2), 276–280.

Oudhia, P. (1995). Traditional knowledge about medicinal insects, mites and spiders in Chattisgarh, India. *Insect Environment, 4*, 57–58.

Padam, G., Chaurasia, O. P., Singh, B., & Attery, D. P. (2000). Medico-botanical survey of Sapi valley of Kargil (Ladakh Himalayas). *Bulletin Medico Ethno Botanical Research, 21*(1 and 2), 1–10.

Panday, H. P. (2004). Seed fume of solanum surattense: A traditional panacea for teeth and gums. *Indian Journal of Traditional Knowledge, 3*(2), 206–207.

Pant, S. C., & Pandey, G. (1995). Ethno-botanical studies on medicinal flora in Tharu tribal pockets in Kumaon region in Uttar Pradesh. *Bulletin Medico Ethno Botanical Research, 16*(1&2), 1–120.

Pant,S. S., & Samant, S. S. (2010). *Ethnobotanical Leaflets 14*, 193–217. Retrieved in February 2013.

Perinchery, A. (2013). History of Indian healing traditions: A science and society initiative. Retrieved March 2013, from http://news.ncbs.res.in/story/history-indian-healing-traditions

Phondani, P. C., Maikhuri, R. K., Rawat, L. S., Farooquee, N. A., Kala, C. P., Vishvakarma, S. C. R., et al. (2010). *Ethnobotanical uses of plants among the Bhotiya tribal communities of Niti valley in Central Himalaya*. India: Ethnobotany Journal. 8.

Rawat, D. S., & Kharwal, A. D. (2011). Traditional phyto-remedies for gynecological complaints in 'Balh Valley', District Mandi (Himachal Pradesh), India. *Ethnobotanical Leaflets, 16*, 546–550.

Rokaya, M. B., Münzbergová, Z. & Timsina, B. (2010). Ethnobotanical study of medicinal plants from the Humla district of western Nepal. *Journal of Ethnopharmacology, 130*: *3*(9): 485–504.

Sajem, A. L., & Gosai, K. (2006). Traditional use of medicinal plants by the Jaintia tribes in North Cachar Hills district of Assam, Northeast India. *Journal of Ethno-biology and Ethno-medicine, 2*, 33. doi:10.1186/1746-4269-2-33.

Samal, P. K., Shah, A., Tiwari, S. C., & Agrawal, D. K. (2004). Indigenous healthcare practices and their linkages with bio-resource conservation and socio-economic development in central Himalayan Region of India. *Indian Journal of Traditional Knowledge, 3*(1), 12–26.

Sand, B. N. & Badola, D. P. (1987).An Ethno-botanical study of J & K State of North-West Himalaya. *Bulletin Medico Ethno Botanical Research, 8* (3&4), 147–154.

Shah, A., Abass, G., & Sharma, M. P. (2012). Ethnobotanical study of some medicinal plants from Tehsil Budhal, District Rajouri, Jammu and Kashmir. *International Multidisciplinary Research Journal, 2*(6), 05–06.

Sharma, P. K., Sethi, G. S., Sharma, S. K., & Sharma, T. K. (2006). Ethno-medicinal observations among the inhabitants of cold desert area of Himachal Pradesh. *Indian Journal of Traditional Knowledge, 5*(3), 358–361.

Srivastava, T. N., & Kapahi, B. K. (1991). Resource survey of plants of potential economic value of Sikkim Himalayas. *Bulletin Medico Ethno Botanical Research, 12*(1–2), 1–11.

Srivastava, T. N., Badola, D. P., Shah, D. C., & Gupta, O. P. (1984). Ethno-medico-botanical exploration of Gurez Valley Kashmir. *Bulletin Medico Ethno Botanical Research, 5*(1& 2), 15–54.

Srivastava, T.N., Kapahi, B.K. & Sarin, Y.K. (1991). Ethno-botanical studies in Lahul and Spiti, Himachal Pradesh. *Ancient Science of Life, 11 3*(4), 126–130.

Tamuli, P., & Saikia, R. (2004). Ethno-medico-botany of the Zeme Tribe of North Cachar Hills district of Assam. *Indian Journal of Traditional Knowledge, 3*(4), 437–441.

Tiwari, J. K., Dangwal, L. R., Rana, C. S., Tiwari, P., & Ballabha, R. (2010). Indigenous uses of plant species in Nanda Devi biosphere reserve, Uttarakhand. *India Report and Opinion, 2*(2), 58–61.

Unnikrishnan, E. (2004). Materia Medica of the Local Health Traditions of Payyannur. Retrieved February 2013, from http://www.cds.ac.in/krpcds/publication/downloads/80.pdf

Wangchuk, P., Pyne, S. G., & Keller, P. A. (2011). Ethnobotanical authentication and identification of Khrog-sman (Lower elevation medicinal plants) of Bhutan. *Journal of Ethnopharmacology, 134*(3), 813–823. doi:10.1016/j.jep.2011.01.034.

Chapter 3
Ethnic Food as Medicament

> *Medicine is not healthcare. Food is healthcare. Medicine is sick care. Let's all get this straight for a change...*
>
> Sidney R Garfield

Abstract The idea of 'food as medicament' is deep-rooted in the primitive therapeutic traditions of all societies. Food habits are the ways in which individuals or communities, in response to the social and cultural stresses select, eat and use available foods. The North-Western Himalayas having wide range of physical, cultural and economic conditions offers a diversity of diet preferences. The communities have evolved local methods of farming, post-harvest management, storage and preservation, food consumption and health care. People living in North-Western Himalayas have developed their own adaptive mechanisms to cope up with the adverse conditions and even the food is preferred keeping in view its nutritive value, 'hot' and 'cold' nature and curative properties. In Himalayan region, most rural communities depend on natural resources comprising of wild edibles and traditional food crops to meet their food requirements mainly during the food crisis and for extra nutritional supplements. This not only offers variety in family diet, but also adds to the household food security. Besides acting as healing foods, the food in the Himalayan region is labor-saving and suitable for large-scale cookery.

Keywords Ethnic food · Medicament · Food habits · Culinary traditions · Traditional food · Food consumption pattern · Traditional crops · Wild edibles · Nutritive and medicinal value

The concept of 'food as medicament' is entrenched in the primeval healing traditions of every civilization. While peeping through the history, one gets to know that the hunter-gatherer ancestors of man probably discovered the curative properties of herbs by viewing the animals who consciously consume some plants to get rid of body ailments. All through the history of medicine, the food and medicine can never be detached. The significance of food reverberates in all conventional systems of healing, including the Indian System of Medicine called, *Ayurveda*. In the most revered and recognized medical texts of *Ayurveda*, the

P. Gupta et al., *Healing Traditions of the Northwestern Himalayas*,
SpringerBriefs in Environmental Science, DOI: 10.1007/978-81-322-1925-5_3,

Charaka Samhita, one finds the progression of rudimentary farming systems from nomadic lifestyle. *Punarvasu Atreya* in *Charaka Samhita* says "It is the nourishing use of food that promotes the health of a person and that which is noxious results in disease". Food thus, not only plays the role of fulfilling the nutritional need of the body, but also helps in maintaining good health. The presence of vital nutrients in the food determines the growth, health and efficiency of a community, the physical and mental well-being of individuals as well as of nations.

> ...Food consumption patterns or food habits are the ways in which individuals or communities, in response to the social and cultural pressures prefer, consume and utilize available foods...

Scientists such as Malinowsky (1944) and Richards (1939) pointed out that body's need for food has done much to mould the society through all activities linked with food production, distribution and consumption. Food is considered as a part of culture that is essential, connected with different kinds of behaviour, and considerably meaningful. Counihan (2000) wrote:

> ...Examination of food ways in all cultures reveals much about power relations, the shaping of community and personality, the construction of family, communication and conception of sex, sexuality and gender...

Farming and rearing of animals started in the last 10,000 years or so. Humans today are the result of what the primeval ancestors ate during their evolutionary journey from scavengers to skilled hunters and from food gatherers to food growers. Archaeological sites have thrown light on the issues of diet, whereas analysis of human remains has helped in explaining the aspects of nutrition. The variety of food preparation across the globe gives an indication of innumerable dietary, aesthetic, agricultural, fiscal, cultural and sacred considerations. Most traditions have an intelligible gastronomy—a precise set of cooking mores, references and practices. While some foods are consumed without preparation, many foods are cooked for reasons of security, scrumptiousness or taste. The term "cooking" encompasses a vast range of techniques, utensils and blending of ingredients to improve the flavor or digestibility of food. It usually requires the choice, measurement and mixing of ingredients in a well-planned *modus operandi.* It may also involve mixing, heating or cooling, boiling, steaming, pressure cooking, fermentation, etc. The culinary tradition of India is as prosperous and assorted as its civilization. This tradition, which is the integral part of Indian Culture, is an art which has been passed on from generation to generation entirely by a word of mouth. History of food reveals the spreading of plants and animals, farming systems, food preferences and taboos together with the ways of cooking and serving. The cultural folklore throughout the history has ascribed the curative or harmful properties of certain foods. This affinity has not vanished with the arrival of science of nutrition and medicine. Even today the food folklore persists, though in many cases it is contradictory with scientific evidence.

3.1 Culinary Traditions of the North-Western Himalayas

Food is indispensable for human existence; however, the attitudes towards food differ across societies, cultures and even individuals. Food, for indigenous societies, is the very first medicine. A number of aspects govern the food consumption patterns; these include social status, religious connotation, habit, knowledge, cultural practices and understanding of its relationship with the wellbeing.

The occurrence of extreme weather conditions such as storms, floods, avalanches, etc., affects the nutrition situation and in turns the health status of Himalayan communities. People living in the remote areas of North-Western Himalayas have developed their own adaptive mechanisms to cope up with the adverse conditions. Thus, the food is preferred keeping in view its nutritive value, 'hot' and 'cold' nature and curative properties. In addition to this, communities have evolved local methods of farming, post-harvest management, storage and preservation, food consumption and health care.

The accessibility of foodstuff depends on the climatic conditions which sequentially have an effect on the farming, availability of natural resources such as fuel-wood, water, soil, etc. and consecutively the life of the communities. Since people living in the North-Western Himalayas practice both agriculture and horticulture, the two act as a good source of food and earnings. Himalayas have diverse agro-climatic conditions and hence different types of crops are grown, which vary from cereals, pulses, oil seeds, and vegetables to subtropical fruits and temperate fruits, besides nut crops. The seasonal cash crops are not adequate to meet the whole year demand and many crops cannot be grown in a particular area, therefore the communities remain dependant on local market for buying foodstuff besides obtaining the same from their own land. People rear livestock for getting wool, milk and meat. Additionally, innumerable wild edibles are also collected and consumed seasonally for their exceptional flavour and medicinal value. In the discussion that follows, an effort has been made to catch a glimpse of the ethnic food and its role as a medicament.

The North-Western Himalayas having wide range of physical, cultural and economic conditions offers a variety of diet preferences which not only vary with demographic and economic conditions, but also differ from village to village exhibiting distinct provincial dietary patterns. Every society frames and elaborates rules regarding the preparation and consumption of food and Himalayan society is no exception to this. Himalayan culture has food habits and traditions well-suited to the survival of communities in particular settings. Which plants and animals are consumed as foodstuff, varies with each culture and society; and what is eaten, how it is prepared, how it is served, who eats it, helps in knowing the functioning of a society. Certain foods are associated with specific groups and the food of a region can also be related with its climate and terrain.

The Himalayan food is different from the rest of the country not only in flavour but also in cooking techniques. It exhibits a perfect blend of diverse cultures and ages. The traditional food of North-Western Himalayas is highly valued for its remarkable use of traditional crops, herbs and condiments. The food consumption patterns vary within different Himalayan states. The food consumption pattern differs is each agro-ecological zone, for instance, in the mid-hills, maize and buttermilk are the main food items, which are consumed throughout the year; in addition to this the consumption of non-vegetarian food is also widespread. The average traditional kitchen makes use of all sorts of meat, pulses and cereal preparations; however, there may be local disparities. In the cold deserts of *Kinnaur* and *Lahaul-Spiti*, there is more stress on utilization of locally cultivated coarse grains like buckwheat, millet, barley, etc. In areas with pastoral traditions, milk and its products are freely utilized in food preparation. In lower areas, the everyday meal consists of rice and pulses or wheat bread and vegetables. Special food is cooked during the festive time. *Dham*—a customary festive meal is cooked only by the traditional chefs or locally called *botis*, and is served on handmade leaf plates. The classic menu for a festive occasion consists of rice, curries cooked in yoghurt, a sour and a *sweet dish*. The customs, rituals and beliefs practiced by communities depict their simple lifestyle and immediacy with nature. Food not only reflects the typical mountain culture but is an important element of life and thus determines the lifestyle of mountain communities.

The food in the North-Western Himalayas is cooked using a variety of methods and thus acquires different tastes and appearances. A number of combinations are used for preparing foods so as to give a variety to the food. Yoghurt and buttermilk is added to a large number of dishes. Almost all the *madharas*[1] are cooked in yoghurt or curd. This is done so precisely or the yoghurt will separate. To avoid this, yoghurt is added and stirred well between each addition. Salt is added at later stage to avoid separation of yoghurt. In order to thicken the gravy of curries, gram flour or maize flour is used along with yoghurt. Tomatoes and spice pastes are prepared by grinding ginger, garlic and onion.

Spices and aromatic plant parts having distinctive flavors and aromas are used in food preparation. While spices are added as flavoring agents, many spices and their oils are believed to possess antimicrobial and antioxidant properties. Spices are used as flavorants or as seasoning both in the fresh and dried form. Most of these are grown locally and used widely. The various spices used are *Ferula asafetida*, *Piper nigrum*, *Capsicum frutescens*, *Coriandrum sativum*, *Brassica sp.*, *Myristica fragrans*, *Eletaria cardmomum*, *Syzygium aromaticum*, *Zingiberofficinale*, *Curcuma longa*, *Cinnamomum aromaticum*, *Trigonella foenum*, *Foeniculum vulgare*, *Allium cepa*, *Allium sativum* and *Cuminum cyminum*. *Cinnamomum aromaticum*, *Foeniculum vulgare*, *Syzygium aromaticum* and *Curcuma longa* are also used in the preparation of traditional deserts.

Along with spices, dry fruits such as *Cocos Nucifera*, dried *Vitis vinifera*, *Phoenix dacty*, *Prunus amygdalus*, *Prunus armenica*, powder of *Mangifera indica*, seeds of *Punica granatum*, seeds of cucumber, watermelon and muskmelon, fruit of *Juglans regia*, *Sesamum indicum* seeds, *Cannabis sativa* seeds, leaves of

---

[1] *Madhara* is the traditional curry cooked in clarified butter and curd.

*Murraya koenigi*and *Ocimum canum, Papaver Somniferum* seeds are used in the preparation of ethnic food. Use of *Brassica juncea*, preferably in sour dishes, is quite common.

Certain foods and drink are taboo in every society, i.e. people abstain from consuming them for religious or cultural reasons. Some authorities impose cultural food taboos in the form of law. The concept of 'hot' and 'cold' has prevailed in Indian culture. From competent doctors, herbalists, folk healers to the general masses, all have reliance and belief in the 'hot' and 'cold' effects of foods. In Himalayan region, pregnancy is believed to be a 'hot' condition and women work until labor starts. There are wide ranges of food, which are considered useful or unsafe among different communities residing in the region. The concept of avoiding 'hot' food is due to the fact that such food items result in premature delivery, miscarriage, or abortion. However, the communities also believe that cold food may cause cold and cough to the mother and infant.

There are a number of restrictions which are followed while preparing, serving and consuming food. These practices are still followed in tribal and non-tribal areas although to a lesser extent. Some of the practices are good while others may not be, for instance, the chef cannot taste the food while preparing it and water is not sipped from tumbler but is poured into the mouth from top because contact of tumbler with mouth is believe to pollute the same. Women cannot enter kitchen and cook food during the menstrual cycle. There are practices which are considered good, as the chef is allowed to go into the kitchen only after taking bath because of the popular belief that food prepared after bathing is as pure as food cooked for holy feast. Thus, such practices not only maintain the sanctity of the kitchen but are healthy in the sense that these keep in mind the essential aspects of hygiene and cleanliness.

Consumption of food in standing or lying position is considered bad. Before serving meal to the family, it is offered to the God and even to the fire in the hearth. A portion of food is kept for a cow, a dog and a crow because of religious beliefs. Only the right hand is used for eating food. There are certain foods and pulses which are eaten only on specific days of a week or a month, for instance, days are marked for the consumption of pulses, *Lens culimaris* is consumed on Tuesday, *Vigna radiata* on Wednesday, *Cicer arietinum* on Thursday, and *Cicer arietinum* or *Vigna radiata* on Saturday. This all is done because of the belief that consuming specific pulses on these days control the planetary effects. *Vigna radiata* is cooked on festive occasions and even on *samkranti.*[2] Such practices provide a variety to the routine food and also constitute a balanced diet. Consumption of *Vigna radiata* or mixed pulses is restricted on festive occasions because of the popular belief that *Vigna radiata* is meant for patients. People

[2] *Samkranti* means transmigration of the Sun from one zodiac constellation to the next. Each *Sakranti* is marked as the beginning of a month in the sidereal solar calendars.

Table 3.1 Food consumption pattern during pregnancy

Number	Name of the food item	Reason
Restricted food items		
1.	Fruits: unripe papaya and mangoes	Considered 'hot' and acts as abortifacient
2.	Pulses: *Dolichos biflorus*	
3.	Cereals: Paspalum *scrobiculatum*	
4.	Vegetables: *Cucurbita pepo, Artocarpus heterophyllus, Amaranthus spinosus, Chenopodium ambrisoides*	
5.	Spices: *Capsicum frutescens*	Affects the eyes of developing fetus
	Decoction of *Carum copticum*	Considered 'hot' and acts as abortifacient
	Dried powder of *Zingiberofficinale*	Considered 'hot' acts as abortifacient. Not given during initial months of pregnancy, but given at the time of parturition
	Seeds of *Brassica juncea*	Considered 'hot' acts as abortifacient
6.	Dry fruits: *Juglans regia,* Phoenixsylvestris, *Prunus dulcis* (during the initial months of pregnancy)	Considered 'hot' and induce abortion Consumption of Phoenix sylvestris is believed to cause difficulty during parturition
7.	Clarified butter (during the initial months of pregnancy)	Considered 'hot' may result in nausea and vomiting
Special food items included		
1.	*Seera*	Considered 'cold' and prevent abortion
2.	Dried powder of *Zingiber officinale* (with the commencement of the 9th month)	For providing strength and considered 'hot' thus give warmth and facilitate easy parturition
3.	Fat rich diet (with the commencement of the 9th month)	For imparting strength and considered 'hot' thus providing heat required by the body for delivery
4.	Seeds of *Piper nigurum* mixed in clarified butter for 9 days (with the commencement of 9th month)	For blood purification of mother
5.	Decoction of *anethum graveolens* seeds mixed with clarified putter (after the completion of gestation period)	Labor induction and facilitate easy parturition
6.	Almonds boiled in milk (after gestation period is over)	Labor induction and facilitate easy parturition

restrict consumption of rice on *Ekadashi*[3]; similarly non-vegetarian food is not consumed during auspicious days. Widows are abstained from consuming non-vegetarian food, *Raphanus sativus, Brassica rapa, Allium cepa, Allium sativum* and *Solanum melongena.*

[3] *Ekadashi* is the eleventh lunar day of the bright or dark fortnight of every lunar month in the Hindu calendar.

Social taboos prevalent in Himalayan society prohibit expectant mothers to consume certain foods. Some of the restricted food items during pregnancy are listed below. Most of these food items are considered 'hot' and thus believe to act as abortifacient. Fruits like unripe papaya, mangoes, pulses as *Dolichos biflorus*, vegetables, pumpkin, jackfruit, *Amaranthus*, *Chenopodium*, spices, dry fruits, like walnuts, almonds, etc. are restricted during pregnancy because of popular belief that they being 'hot' in nature may result in a miscarriage (Table 3.1).

On the other hand, a few foodstuffs are specially recommended during pregnancy. Some of them are restricted in the initial months of pregnancy, but can be a part of the diet in the later stages. These may include milk and milk products, dry fruits and clarified butter. A few ethnic delicacies for instance, *paraks, gheyor, arsay, bhalay, bathuru,* etc. are fed to the expectant mothers. Ceremonial occasions are marked to feed special food to the pregnant woman. This is usually done between seventh and the 9th month. Parents or relatives prepare special food of choice for an expectant mother and feed her the same. Powder of *Piper nigurum* seeds mixed in clarified butter is given to the expectant mother for blood purification. Even the *anethum graveolens* seeds are given during the initial months of pregnancy. With the commencement of 9th month, pregnant lady is given dried powder of *Zingiber officinale*, clarified butter; almonds boiled in milk and clarified butter mixed with milk. Certain "hot foods" which are restricted in the initial months are given in the 9th month to provide warmth and energy to the body which is required after parturition.

Some of these practices are not good, such as, restriction on fruits, fat rich diet and dry fruits as this not only affect the nutritional status of mothers but often affect the health of developing embryo. Initiation of healthy food in the latter stage however makes up for the loss to some extent. Not only during pregnancy, but even after delivery, the diet of mother is taken care of. Mixed opinions came into limelight regarding the food of mother after parturition. Some food items are restricted and some others are incorporated as special items into the diet of lactating mothers. This is again based on the concept of 'hot' and 'cold'. There are beliefs that mother's diet has an implication on the health of a child, especially when the mother is breast feeding the child. Consumption of curd or buttermilk, sour food items like, pickles, lemon, chutneys, salt, pulses such as *Vigna radiata*, *Phaseolus vulgaris*, green leafy vegetables, *Cucurbita pepo, Abelmoschus esculentus, Solanum melongena* and all kinds of fruits, is restricted during the first few months of lactation. This is done because of the belief that these items, being 'cold' causes in cough and cold in the infants or may cause diarrhea and abdominal pains. A few food items are introduced in the regular diet of lactating mothers to provide energy and to enhance adequate secretion of breast milk. These acts as galactogogue and include water of boiled rice, sugary foods, *Lens culimaris*, fried in *Cuminum cyminum,* salt tea with butter and grinded walnuts, clarified butter and animal fat. Intake of sugary food is believed to augment the secretion of breast milk, whereas intake of salt lessens it. Consumption of salty food is restricted for

Table 3.2 Food consumption pattern of a lactating mother

Number	Name of the food item	Reason
Restricted food items		
1.	Curd /buttermilk	Considered 'cold' and thus cause cough and cold in the newly born baby
2.	Sour food, as pickles, lemon, chutneys	Considered 'cold' and hence cause cough and cold in new born infant. It is believe to affect mother's body resulting in body aches
3.	Salt	Inhabits adequate secretion of breast milk
4.	Rice (in district Kinnaur)	Considered 'cold' and hence capable of causing in cold to new born.
5.	Maize bread	Considered 'heavy'
6.	Pluses: *Vigna mungo, Cicer Arietinum, Phaseolus aureus*	Diarrhea and colic pain in the child
7.	Vegetables: green leafy vegetables, *Cucurbita pepo, Abelmoschus esculentus, Solanum melongena, Brassica oleracea*	Diarrhea and colic pain in the child
8.	All fruits for first few months	Considered 'cold' and may result in cough and cold in new born
Special food items included		
1.	Rice water	Acts as galactogogue
2.	Sweet food mainly rice pudding (rice boiled in milk) Sweet rice (rice cooked in molasses/ jaggery)	Acts as galactogogue
3.	*Kasayatu chawal*	Considered 'hot' and good for mother and child
4.	*Lens culimaris* fried in *Cuminum cyminum*	Acts as galactogogue
5.	Salt tea (in Kinnaur) with butter and grinded walnuts	Acts as galactogogue
6.	Clarified butter and animal fat	Considered 'hot' and thus believed to provide heat and strength to the body of both mother and child. Gargles of melted fat are recommended after delivery for importing strength to the teeth which are believed to become week after delivery
7.	Dried powder of *Zingiber officinale* fried in clarified butter	Considered 'hot' thus provide heat for the body of both mother and child
8.	Dry fruits boiled in milk	Considered 'hot' thus provide warmth and strength to the body of both mother and infant
9.	*Seera*	Though considered 'cold' but given along with preparation of *Zingiberofficinale* to counterbalance the excessive warmth if produced due to the consumption of *Zingiberofficinale*
10.	Milk consumption three to four times	Acts as galactogogue

Table 3.3 List of foods restricted or prescribed for common body discomforts

Number	Name of the disorder	Restricted food items	Prescribed food items
1.	Acne and skin disorders	'Hot', greasy and spicy foods, including molasses, jaggery, sugary foods	Oral administration of paste of *Piper nigrum* in clarified butter, decoction of *Azadirachta indica* leaves
2.	Arthritis	'Cold' and sour food in addition to rice, pulses, whole grains, Colocasia *esculenta*, *Solanum tuberosum*, etc.	Intake of *Linum usitatissimum* seeds, pudding of *Aloe barbadensis*
3.	Cold	'Cold' and sour food items, for instance, curd, buttermilk, *Citrullis lanatus*, *Citrus sinensis*, *Citrus limon*, cold water	'Hot' food items as soup of *Cicer arietinum*. Pudding of chickpea flour cooked in milk
4.	Cough	Milk, fat rich foods, for instance, walnut, groundnut, clarified butter in addition to 'Cold' and sour food items	Decoction of *Viola odorata*, paste of *Pistacia integerrima* fruit in honey
5.	Dyspepsia	'Hot', greasy and spicy foods	Decoction of *Mentha longifolia*, chutney of *Punica granatum* seeds, *Mentha longifolia and* rhododendron flowers
6.	Fever	'Cold' and sour food items, for instance, curd, buttermilk, *Citrullis lanatus*, *Citrus sinensis*, *Citrus limon*	Dish of rice and legumes
7.	Nasal bleeding	'Hot' and spicy foods	'Cold' and sour food items, for instance, curd, buttermilk, watermelon, orange, lemon, cold water, squash of rhododendron flowers
8.	Stomachache	'Cold' and sour food in addition to Colocasia *esculenta*, *Solanum tuberosum*, *Cucurbita pepo*, curd, buttermilk	Decoction of *Bunium persicum*

16 days after delivery, as it prevents the adequate secretion of milk. Dried powder of *Zingiber officinale* rhizome fried in clarified butter and dry fruits boiled in milk are given to lactating mothers. *Seera* prepared from wheat grains is considered highly nutritious and hence fed once a day. Milk is given to the lactating mothers three to four times. Thus, the food taboos have not only shaped the food consumption patterns of communities, but also have implications on health status of people (Table 3.2).

In addition to the restricted diet that a woman is given during pre-natal and post-natal period, a number of foods are restricted or prescribed for common body discomforts. Some of these are shown in Table 3.3.

In the Himalayan region, most rural communities depend on natural resources including wild edibles and traditional food crops to meet their food requirements particularly during the food crisis and for extra nutritional supplements. This not only offers diversity in family diet, but also adds to the household food security. The traditional food crops and wild edibles offer healthy options to highly processed foodstuff and pharmaceuticals, thereby improving health status of Himalayan communities. Wild fruits are important sources of minerals, fibre, vitamins, and provide vital nutrients required for healthy living. Additionally, it has been recognized that wild fruits have the so-called 'anti-nutritional' factors which can diminish the nutrient bioavailability, especially if these are present in larger quantity. On the other hand, scientific studies have shown that the anti-nutritional factors could prevent and treat several diseases. The most important nutrients present in wild edibles and traditional crops are: carbohydrates, in form of starch and free sugars; oils, proteins, minerals, ascorbic acid, and antioxidant phenols. Plants, possessing phyto-chemicals with antioxidant activity, have caught the attention of scientific community in the recent years. Antioxidants, which restrain the oxidation of organic molecules, are essential, not only in food preservation, but also in providing resistance to body against oxidative stress. Dietary fiber (DF) on the other hand, plays an important role in diminishing the risks of constipation, diabetes, cardiovascular diseases, diverticulosis and obesity. Wild edibles and traditional crops are the only sources of dietary fiber. Diet of Himalayan people mainly consist of a variety of plant foods such as cereals, pulses, green leafy vegetables, wild edibles as roots, tubers, vegetables, oil seeds, spices and condiments. Wild edibles are consumed in fresh or dried form. The polysaccharides constituting the major part of dietary fiber in wild edibles and traditional crops are useful for body, since its consumption decreases the plasma cholesterol levels.

Traditionally grown crops and wild edibles in North Western Himalayas have nutritive and curative value. Because of the curative properties, they possess, these are consumed both seasonally and occasionally. Some of these having curative properties are even given to the patients suffering from various bodily discomforts. A few among these are:

Vernacular name of plant	**Chulai**
Botanical name	*Amaranthus spinosus* L.
Part used	Leaves, stem and seeds
Usage pattern	Leaves cooked as vegetable and seeds are used for preparing bread
People's perception	Owing to its easy digestibility, it is traditionally fed to the patients who are improving from ill health or fasting period. The leaf juice being 'hot' is used to relieve chest congestion

(continued)

(continued)

Nutritive and medicinal value	It has a high nutritional value because of the presence of essential micronutrients, vitamin C, iron, phosphorous, magnesium and calcium more than what is found in animal products. The plant is particularly rich in lysine, and essential amino acids that are usually lacking in cereal based diets. Its seed contain more protein than other grains such. The plant has been found to be effective in combating diseases including diabetes and cardiovascular diseases (Kirtikar and Basu 1993)
Vernacular name of plant	**Ogla**
Botanical name	*Fagopyrum tataricum* (L.) Gaertn.
Part used	Seeds
Usage pattern	Flour of buckwheat is used for making ethnic foods such as *chilare, chilta, lapphi,* etc.
People's perception	Easily digestible and highly nutritious
Nutritive and medicinal value	Complementary to cereal flour, and can be used to improve their nutritional quality, as it contain essential amino acids. It has numerous health benefits such as anti-hyperglycemic effect, hypotensive activity, anti-oxidative properties, hypocholesterolemic effect and anticancer activity (Tomotake et al. 2001; Kawa et al. 2003)
Vernacular name of plant	**Bathu**
Botanical name	Chenopodium album L.
Part used	Leaves and seeds
Usage pattern	The seeds are boiled to make gruel or sweet pudding. Parched seeds along with molasses/jaggery are fed to the children
People's perception	The seeds being 'hot' are considered abortifacient. Powdered seeds are given to children to treat intestinal worms. Parched seeds are given during the chickenpox
Nutritive and medicinal value	Useful in cold, general weakness and purgative. Its seeds contain whole set of essential amino acids. It has higher lysine content. Its leaves are good source of high-quality protein concentrate (Kumar and Kumar 2008)
Vernacular name of Plant	**Koda**
Botanical name	Paspalum *scrobiculatum* L.
Part used	Seeds
Usage pattern	Seeds used for preparing traditional bread
People's perception	The seeds being 'hot', are considered abortifacient
Nutritive and medicinal value	It acts as appetizer, astringent, digestive, diuretic, emollient, refrigerant, and stomachic. Its seeds are rich in vitamins, especially niacin, B6 and folacin, calcium, iron, potassium, magnesium, and zinc. *Paspalum scrobiculatum* is traditionally used to treat diabetes mellitus (Jain et al. 2010)

(continued)

(continued)

Vernacular name of plant	**Jau**
Botanical name	*Hordeum vulgare* L.
Part used	Seeds
Usage pattern	Seeds used for preparing traditional dishes like *siddu, vit, sattu, torma,* etc.
People's perception	Considered highly nutritious. Acts as a galactogogue
Nutritive and medicinal value	It has superior nutritional qualities due to the presence of beta-glucan (an anti-cholesterol substance), acetylcholine (a substance which nourishes nervous system) and easy digestibility (due to low gluten contents) besides high lysine, thiamin and riboflavin (Spiller 2001)
Vernacular name of plant	**Makki**
Botanical name	*Zea mays* L.
Part used	Seeds
Usage pattern	Seeds used for preparing leavened bread.
People's perception	Fresh corn silk boiled in water is helpful in curing renal calculi
Nutritive and medicinal value	The health benefits of maize include management of diabetes, prevention of heart ailments and lowering hypertension. It is a rich source of vitamins A, B, E and many minerals. The vitamin B_{12} and folic acid present in seeds help prevent anaemia. Its high fibre content plays a role in preventing constipation, haemorrhoids and colorectal cancer. The corn silk acts as demulcent, diuretic, mild stimulant and vasodilator. It reduces blood sugar levels and used in the treatment of diabetes mellitus (Abdel-Wahab et al. 2002)
Vernacular name of plant	**Kauni**
Botanical name	*Panicum italicum* L.
Part used	Seeds
Usage pattern	Seeds boiled as rice or as porridge
People's perception	Formed the part of staple diet at the time of famine or drought. Its seeds are not attacked by any pests even for a decade
Nutritive and medicinal value	Considered highly nutritive and light diet
Vernacular name of plant	**Kulath**
Botanical name	Dolichos biflorus L.
Part used	Seeds
Usage pattern	Seeds cooked as *dal*, and ethnic food like *indray* and *bhaley* are prepared from its seeds
People's perception	It is believed to possess 'hot' properties and at times, its consumption leads to nausea
Nutritive and medicinal value	The seed is bitter, acrid, hot, dry, astringent to bowels, fattening, anti-helmentic, antipyretic and useful in the treatment of tumours, asthma, bronchitis, hiccup, heart-troubles, disease of brain and eyes, intestinal colic, piles, leucoderma, inflammation, liver troubles, etc.

(continued)

(continued)

Vernacular name of plant	**Chulli**
Botanical name	Prunus armeniaca L.
Part used	Fruit and kernel
Usage pattern	Fruit used for preparing local wine, dried fruit is used for making chutney, puddings and ethnic dishes like *dubti, chulphunting, chuluk*, etc.
People's perception	The dry fruit is believed to have laxative properties. The oil is highly nutritive and has curative effect on aching joints, earache and aching eyes
Nutritive and medicinal value	Its oil supply essential fatty acids such as linoleic and arachidonic acids. Oil is also used for producing drug dispersants in therapeutics. Fresh fruits are a good source of protein, lipid, and fatty acids for human nutrition
Vernacular name of plant	**Anardana**
Botanical name	*Punica granatum* L.
Part used	Seeds
Usage pattern	Seeds used for preparing chutney to treat nausea.
People's perception	Seeds used in preparation of various medicines. Used in home-based medicine to treat sore throats, coughs, digestive disorders, and to expel intestinal worms
Nutritive and medicinal value	It has great nutritional values and numerous health benefits. Effective in the treatment of cancer, osteoarthritis and other diseases
Vernacular name of plant	**Akhroat**
Botanical name	*Juglans regia* L.
Part used	Fruit
Usage pattern	Seed part of the fruit (kernel) is consumed fresh, while dried fruit is the ingredient of number of ethnic foods
People's perception	Extract of its stem bark is used for treating inflammation in foot. Stem bark is used for cleaning teeth
Nutritive and medicinal value	Nuts are nutrient-rich food because of high contents of fats, proteins, vitamins and minerals. These are good source of flavonoids, sterols and related polyphenols. They possess antibacterial, antifungal, antiviral and antioxidant activity (Upadhyay et al. 2010a, b)
Vernacular name of plant	**Til**
Botanical name	*Sesamum indicum* L.
Part used	Seeds
Usage pattern	Seeds are grinded and added as flavorants in many ethnic foods such as *siddu, bedi,* chutney, etc.
People's perception	Considered 'hot', regular application of seed oil on joints like knee, elbow and shoulder helps in treating arthritis
Nutritive and medicinal value	Sesame seeds have anti-cancer properties due to the presence of sesamin and sesamolin besides offering protection against cardiovascular system diseases and disorders

(continued)

(continued)

Vernacular name of plant	**Bhang**
Botanical name	*Cannabis sativa* L.
Part used	Seeds locally named as *Bhangolu*
Usage pattern	Seeds are ingredient of number of ethnic foods, for instance curries, *siddu, bedi*, etc.
People's perception	Considered 'hot' and usually consumed during the winter season. Excessive consumption often leads to nausea, vomiting and headache
Nutritive and medicinal value	Possesses diuretic, anti-emetic, anti-epileptic, anti-inflammatory, painkilling and antipyretic properties (Lozano 2001)
Vernacular name of plant	**Gandela**
Botanical name	Murraya koenigii L.
Part used	Leaves
Usage pattern	Used as flavouring agent in curries, stem used for cleaning teeth
People's perception	Its consumption keeps one fresh and healthy It is good for heart problems. Regular intake of its leaves is good for general health
Nutritive and medicinal value	Carbazole alkaloids present in the leaves, fruits, roots and bark of this plant have anti-diabetic, anticancer, antibacterial and antioxidant properties (Bhandari 2012)
Vernacular name of plant	**Phabari**
Botanical name	*Ocimum canum* L.
Part used	Leaves
Usage pattern	Leaves added as flavoring agent and condiment in curries and chutneys
People's perception	Effective in gastric problems
Nutritive and medicinal value	Considered as antibacterial, antifungal, antispasmodic, digestive, expectorant, stimulant, stomachic etc. The plant is generally used in the treatment of problems concerning digestion and nervous system (Prakash and Gupta 2005)
Vernacular name of plant	**Affim-dana**
Botanical name	*Papaver somniferum* L.
Part used	Seeds
Usage pattern	Seeds are ingredient in number of ethnic foods, for instance curries, *siddu, bedi*, etc.
People's perception	Considered 'hot' and usually consumed during the winter season
Nutritive and medicinal value	It acts as analgesic and induce sedation and cough depression

(continued)

(continued)

Vernacular name of plant	**Rai**
Botanical Name	*Brassica juncea* L.
Part used	Seeds
Usage pattern	Leaves cooked as vegetable. Oil is extracted from its seeds. Seeds are used as flavouring agent and are also pickled. Grinded seed powder is dissolved in buttermilk and consumed after 3–4 h
People's perception	Seeds used for treating worm infestation
Nutritive and medicinal value	Effective in arthritis, foot-ache and rheumatism. Seeds are used in the treatment of abscesses, colds and stomach disorders (Grover et al. 2002)
Vernacular name of plant	**Churo**
Botanical name	*Euphorbia royleana* Boiss.
Part used	Stem
Usage pattern	It is cooked in form of vegetable. It is used to prepare nuggets
People's perception	Latex effectively treats digestive disorders and insect bites
Nutritive and medicinal value	Plant has high medicinal properties and its latex in small doses acts as a purgative (Singh and Singh 2012)
Vernacular name of plant	**Kawar-pattha**
Botanical name	*Aloe* barbadensis Mill
Part used	Leaf
Usage pattern	It is cooked as vegetable and also pickled. It is used for medicinal purpose and is given to diabetic patient
People's perception	Considered 'hot' and effective in treating aching joints
Nutritive and medicinal value	Antioxidant, fungicidal, controls diabetes and cholesterol
Vernacular name of plant	**Ramban**
Botanical name	*Agave Americana* L.
Part used	Leaves and floral stalk
Usage pattern	Stalk is cooked as vegetable in the month of March and is believe to cure digestive disorders. Its extract is dropped in ear to cure ear ache
People's perception	Considered 'hot' and act as abortifacient
Nutritive and medicinal value	It is used in preparation of various *Ayurvedic* medicines
Vernacular name of plant	**Lingru**
Botanical name	*Diplazium esculentum* Retz.
Part used	Immature fronds
Usage pattern	Cooked as vegetable in the month of April–May. In some areas fronds are pickled for long-term usage
People's perception	Considered as healthy and nutritious
Nutritive and medicinal value	Contain Beta-carotene, vitamin E, riboflavin, ascorbic acid, calcium. Both fresh and boiled leaves have anti-oxidative activities higher than alpha-tocopherol

(continued)

(continued)

Vernacular name of plant	**Sonth**
Botanical name	*Zingiber officinale*
Part used	Rhizome
Usage pattern	Its extract mixed with honey is used for treating cold and cough. Its dried powder, fried in clarified butter is given to mothers after delivery
People's perception	Powder is considered 'hot' and used in preparing number of decoctions meant for treating various diseases
Nutritive and medicinal value	Medically ginger is used as a stimulant and carminative and is used frequently for dyspepsia and colic. It relieves joint pain from arthritis (Al-Amin 2006)
Vernacular name of plant	**Chuchh**
Botanical name	Nasturtium officinale L.
Part used	Leaves
Usage pattern	Leaves cooked as vegetable
People's perception	Considered hot and useful in body aches
Nutritive and medicinal value	Many benefits for its consumption are claimed, such as that it acts as a stimulant, a source of phytochemicals and antioxidants, a diuretic, an expectorant, and a digestive aid
Vernacular name of plant	**Haldi**
Botanical name	*Curcuma longa* L.
Part used	Rhizome
Usage pattern	Rhizome powder is boiled in milk and given during any internal or external injuries. Fresh rhizome is pickled and cooked as vegetable
People's perception	Acts as an anti-inflammatory and relieves body aches and cure internal injuries
Nutritive and medicinal value	The dried rhizome is considered to be stimulating, carminative, purifying, anti-inflammatory and Antihelmentic. Its paste is applied on wounds, bruises, inflammatory problems of joint and sprain
Vernacular name of plant	**Pudina**
Botanical name	Mentha viridis L.
Part used	Leaves
Usage pattern	The leaves are used in chutneys, leaves used as salad, spice
People's perception	Leaf extract is effective in dyspepsia
Nutritive and medicinal value	Effective in digestive problems, including nausea, flatulence and hiccups as it relaxes the stomach muscles. The essential oil, menthol, has analgesic, local anesthetic and counterirritant properties (Shah and Mello 2004)
Vernacular name of plant	**Dhaeu**
Botanical name	*Artocarpus lakoocha* Roxb.
Part used	Fruit
Usage pattern	Fruit cooked as vegetable and also pickled

(continued)

(continued)

People's perception	Considered 'hot' and excessive consumption results in stomach ache
Nutritive and medicinal value	Possess antioxidant constituents helpful in the maintenance of health and protection from coronary heart disease (Pandey and Bhatnaga 2009)
Vernacular name of plant	**Methi**
Botanical name	*Trigonella foenum* L.
Part used	Leaves and seeds
Usage pattern	Leaves cooked as vegetable. Seeds used as flavouring agent and as a condiment
People's perception	Seeds and leaves have property of relieving gastric problem
Nutritive and medicinal value	Fenugreek seed is known to exhibit anti-diabetic properties and effects such as anti-cancer and thyroxine-induced hyperglycaemia (Al-Habori and Raman 2002)
Vernacular name of plant	**Kachnar**
Botanical name	Bauhinia variegate L.
Part used	Buds
Usage pattern	Buds cooked as vegetable and pickled
People's perception	Excessive consumption of its buds leads to gastric problem
Nutritive and medicinal value	Plant used against bronchitis, leprosy, tumours and ulcers
Vernacular name of plant	**Alsi**
Botanical name	*Linum usitatissimum* L.
Part used	Seeds
Usage pattern	Seeds are ingredient of number of ethnic foods, for instance *siddu, bedi*, etc.

Dal is a preparation of pulses, dried lentils, peas or beans which have been stripped of their external hulls and split. It also refers to the thick stew prepared from pulses, a vital component of Indian cuisine. It is regularly consumed with rice and vegetables in south India, and with both rice and wheat-based flat bread throughout the northern region

By making use of one or more of the above ingredients, a number of ethnic dishes are prepared by communities inhabiting the Himalayan region. Some of these have curative and nutritive properties and given in unhealthy or sick condition.

Churra is a traditional form of prepared cheese, usually prepared by using yak milk. It is considered highly nutritious and normally consumed in the breakfast along with tea.

Moddi consists of roasted or parched wheat or soybean grains and thought to be nourishing in anaemia and weakness.

Jhol or *khairu* is prepared from buttermilk and act as good appetizer. It is usually consumed with rice or maize bread. It reduces body heat in summers

Ambua is prepared by using unripe mangoes during the summers. It is served with rice and consumed as taster.

Anardane Ka Mahani is prepared by using dried seeds of *Punica granatum*. It acts as rich source of vitamin C and also believed to cure cough and cold. These seeds are also used to prepare *Anardanae ki chutney*. Leaves of *Mentha viridis* are added to impart flavour to the chutney. It lessens the effect of heat and can be given to sick person without having any side effects.

Khobli is a steamed food mainly prepared in the winter season. Wheat or barley flour, animal fat, salt and spices are the main ingredients. It is served with clarified butter.

Sattu is the grinded flour of parched/ roasted grains of barley or maize. The one prepared from barley is consumed with salt tea or apricot oil, while the one prepared from maize is consumed with buttermilk. It is highly nutritious and ready-to-eat versatile traditional food and is a good source of energy. It requires no cooking before serving, and acts as good source of proteins and given to the children.

Dhu is a boiled food cooked by using maize or barley flour. It is served with clarified butter and jaggery and considered highly nutritive and good source of carbohydrates.

Chawari is instant snack prepared by using dry dates, dry fruits, sugar and consumed with milk. It is given to lactating mothers soon after the delivery.

Gimta is made by using goat's intestine, Ditch Millet's flour, salt and spices. It involves boiling and shallow frying techniques. It is consumed with tea and considered highly nutritive having rich source of proteins and fats.

Chulphanting is prepared from dry apricot, which are soaked overnight and boiled in water, to which salt or sugar is added as per the taste. The gruel so prepared is good source of vitamin C, highly nutritious besides acting as traditional laxative.

Lapphi is cooked by using chenopodium seed, molasses and water. The ingredients are boiled in water and the soup so prepared is served hot along with meals. It is rich source of carbohydrates and proteins; however, the over consumption results in dysentery.

Bari is a semi-solid boiled food prepared by boiling wheat flour in water, to which a pinch of salt is added. The dish is served with clarified butter. Being healthy, it is given to lactating mother soon after delivery.

Shiroltu is a semi-solid mass of dried apricot, which after drying is mashed and consumed with salt and spices. It is eaten for change of taste; used for preparing chutney to impart sour taste to any dish. It is a rich source of vitamin C.

Seera is prepared by making use of wheat or rice grains. Wheat or rice grains are soaked in water for 10–15 days. Water is decanted and soft grains are grinded to form thick paste, which is allowed to dry in sun. *Seera* is fried in clarified butter to which sugar is added. It is highly effective in treating menstrual disorders, especially in the incidence of repeated abortions. It is nutritive and is good source of proteins and carbohydrates. It is given to pregnant women and even lactating mothers. Being nutritious, it is a good supplementary food for children.

Tyaap is a usually consumed during the summers. The fresh rice grains are parched and soaked in milk overnight. The same is consumed in the morning by adding sugar and dry fruits.

Tahelva/ sudka is a traditional health drink prepared by using dry almonds, rice, cucumber seeds, seeds of watermelon and muskmelon, poppy seeds and sugar. The ingredients are grinded, fried in clarified butter, boiled in milk, to which sugar is added. The drink is allowed to cool and served in morning.

Luguru, the rice cooked in the molasses is given to the patients suffering from chickenpox.

Danabath is the traditional variety of red rice boiled in water and fed to the patients of Diarrhoea along with clarified butter and poppy seeds.

Lakarcha has leaves of locally available tea, salt, walnuts, pine seeds and yak butter as main constituents. It is generally consumed in tribal areas and served as bowlfuls. Since butter and salt are the main ingredients, the drink provides ample caloric energy suited to high altitudes. It is believed to prevent chapped lips and dehydration.

Angoori is a local grape wine prepared by using traditional fermentation technique. The drink is effectively used for managing fever and cold.

Peech is the boiled rice water, which is believed to be highly nutritive and instant food given to manage dysentery. It is also given to lactating mothers for increasing the secretion of breast milk.

There are several dietary practices which are designed particularly to protect and promote health. Thus, the knowledge on the dietary practices can help in retaining the positive habits and changing the negative ones. Consumption of protein-rich foods, such as, local variety of *Oryza sp. Fagopyrum tataricum, Triticum acstivum, Zea mays, Paspalum scrobiculatum, Chenopodium album, Phaseolus vulgaris, Vigna radiata, Hordeum vulgare*and *Dolichos biflorus*, etc. is certainly helpful. Another custom frequently found among people is the large intake of buttermilk/ curd rather than milk. The souring of milk has little effect on its nutritive value but to a large extent reduces the number of pathogenic organisms present. In some communities, the living conditions are bad and awareness regarding health and hygiene is also poor. In such families, milking may not be hygienically performed and even the container in which the milk is collected is likely to be contaminated. In such cases, use of buttermilk or curdled milk rather than fresh milk is more beneficial. Communities ferment certain foods before consumption, which improves the nutritional quality and reduces bacterial contamination of the food.

The conventional use of green leafy vegetables and wild edibles is another beneficial practice. The green leafy vegetables are rich sources of carotene, ascorbic acid, iron, calcium etc. and they also contain useful quantities of protein. Non-cultivated or wild edibles such as *Agave americana, Euphorbia royleana, Indigofera pulchella, Bahaunia variegate, Nasturtium officinalis, Diplazium esculentum, Aloe banbadensis,* etc.as well as the cultivated food, such as *Abelmoschus esculentus, Trigonella foenum, Lagenaria vulgaris, Cucurbita pepo, Brassica oleracca, Brassica rapa, Daucus carota, Pisum sativum* are rich in vitamins. Similarly, many wild and cultivated edibles are rich in vitamin C, for instance, *Prunus armenica, Artocarpus lackoocha, Citrus pseudolimon, Punica granatum,* etc. are consumed frequently by the people.

Traditional methods involved in the grain preparation produce more nutritious products than does elaborate machine milling. People still prefer traditional methods of post-harvest management and food processing. Such methods are good and prevent loss of nutrients. Even today, there are traditional grinding mills meant for milling grains. Among various cooking methods, boiling and steaming are quite beneficial as they prevent the loss of important nutrients. People cook sprout legume seeds, which enhances the nutritive value of legumes, as does the soaking of whole-grain cereals before their processing into some ethnic food or alcoholic beverage. These seeds and grains usually have high vitamin B content. Such practices not only provide nutrient rich food but also contribute to good health.

In certain areas, conventional food customs are practiced by a particular group or community, for instance, consumption of non-vegetarian food is restricted by Brahmin community and this restriction may be linked with religion or caste. According to the Hindu school of thought, non-vegetarian food is restricted on certain auspicious days, fasts and some holy week days and people follow such religious directives. They have developed their own reasoning for this. A very good example of this may be sited here. On the auspicious occasion of Shivaratri[4] people usually observe fast and consume only phalahar[5] and the consumption of non-vegetarian food is avoided but people inhabiting certain parts of district Shimla, slaughter goats on this occasion. They have developed their own reasoning and have linked this practice to the religion itself. Another example in this may be sited with regard to the influence of caste. Throughout the region, it was observed that people avoid taking and sharing food with people of lower caste. Even during marriages they are served separately, but, on the contrary during a marriage in a low caste family, Brahmins chefs are invited to cook the food.

The type of occupation also contributes in determining the food habits of people. The *gaddi*tribes, who lead a nomadic life, depend on the availability of wild edibles to meet their food requirements. They have devised ways to cope up with the adverse climatic conditions and situations of non-availability of food. They don't carry much with them and hence make use of locally available wild food. Similarly, the agriculturists prefer consumption of cereals and pulses grown in their own fields.

It was found that several taboos are imposed because the food had on some occasion caused illness or some health problems. A very interesting example is regarding the consumption of wild spinach, locally named as *jalaga*. If the plant is consumed in raw form it causes dysentery. Even the water used for washing the plant, if consumed, causes dysentery, and the same plant if consumed after cooking, cures the problem. While analyzing the culinary customs of Himalayan communities, certain aspects need to be focused with regard to its:

---

[4] *Shivaratri* is the night of Lord Shiva, and is celebrated on the 14th night of *Magha* or *Phalguna* month of the Hindu calendar every year.

[5] *Phalahar is* edibles comprising fruits and items other than cereals/ grains, consumed on the occasion of fast.

Diversity and suitability according to climate: The consumption of salt tea, for example, during the extreme winters not only nourishes the body but also prevents the dehydration or loss of body fluids.

Ingredients: The ethnic food in the Himalayas is mainly prepared from the locally available vegetables, spices, cereals, pulses and wild edibles. The wild edibles have therapeutic properties and besides being nutritious they are apposite substitute for routine foodstuffs. Many of the spices and flavorants used in the recipes are drawn locally, which imparts a unique flavor and aroma to the food. Use of artificial coloring agents, creams, jellies, preservatives is avoided. Many of the food items are prepared using traditional cereals. Use of molasses, jaggery, curd, buttermilk, apricot oil, etc. has numerous health benefits, which must be retained and promoted.The wild edibles collected by people are generally sorted out, cooked or sold in the local markets. The shelf-life of wild edibles is usually very short but people have devised methods to preserve and use harvests in a number of ways.

Use of Indigenous Cookery Technologies: The communities make use of traditional technologies, for instance, fermentation which is practiced for thousands of years has its own advantage. The traditional fermentation of foods enriches the diet by imparting diversity of flavors, aromas and textures in food substrates. Biologically, it enriches the food substrates with protein, essential amino acids, fatty acids and vitamins. Many of the foods are steamed and their consumption is advantageous because steaming preserves the dietary value of food, its color, flavor and aroma. It makes the food lighter and easily digestible. Steaming reduces the risk of overcooking. In many of the delicacies, boiling is used as the way of cooking which not only suits large-scale food preparation and saves fuel but maintains the nutritive stock, color and flavor of food. In case of non-vegetation cooking, boiling loosens the toughness of meat and makes it more appetizing and toothsome.

Thus, besides acting as healing foods, the food in the Himalayan region is labor-saving and suitable for large-scale cookery. Steaming is cost-effective process as low heat is required and a multi-tiered steamer is used besides traditional steaming techniques, which make use of grass, leaves and twigs. Today we notice farm-fresh whole foods being steadily displaced by manufactured duplication. To lessen the nutritional deficiency disorders and to encourage nourishing diets and healthy lifestyles a multi-sectoral approach involving the relevant sectors in societies is required. The food sector figures outstandingly in this endeavor and must be given due importance in support of healthy diet for individuals and population. Food strategies must not simply be directed at ensuring food security for all, but must also realize the consumption of adequate quantities of harmless and quality foods that together make up a healthy diet. Therefore, rather than changing traditional food habits, based on current scientific evidence, valuable lessons may be learnt by tapping the wisdom of ethnic communities by understanding about their food beliefs and how they influence health decision making.

References

Abdel-Wahab, S. M., El-Tanbouly, N. D., Kassem, H. A., & Mohamed, E. A. (2002). Phytochemical and biochemical study of corn silk (styles and stigmas of Zea mays L.). *Bulletin of Faculty of Pharmacy, 40*, 93–102.

Al-Amin, Z. M. (2006). Antidiabetic and hypolipidaemic properties of Zingiber (Zingiber officinale) in streptozotocin-induced diabetic rats. *British Journal of Nutrition, 96*, 660–666.

Al-Habori, M., & Raman, A. (2002). *Pharmacological Properties in Fenugreek—the genus Trigonella* (1st Ed.). by G. A. Petropoulos (Ed.), London: Taylor and Francis.

Bhandari, P. R. (2012). Curry leaf (Murraya koenigii) or cure leaf: Review of its curative properties. *Journal of Medical Nutrition and Nutraceuticals, 1*, 92–97.

Counihan, C. M. (2000). The social and cultural uses of food. In K. F. Kiple, & K. C. Ornelas (Eds.) *The Cambridge world history of food*. Cambridge: Cambridge University Press.

Grover, J. K., Yadav, S., & Vats, V. (2002). Hypoglycemic and anti-hyperglycemic effect of Brassica juncea diet and their effect on hepatic glycogen content and the key enzymes of carbohydrate metabolism. *Molecular and Cellular Biochemistry, 241*(1–2), 95–101.

Jain, S., Bhatia, G., Barik, R., Kumar, P., Jain, A., & Dixit, V. K. (2010). Anti-diabetic activity of Paspalum scrobiculatum L. in alloxan induced diabetic rats. *Journal of Ethnopharmacology, 3, 127*(2), 325–328. doi: 10.1016/j.jep.2009.10.038.

Kawa, J. M., Taylor, C. G., & Ptzybylski, R. (2003). Buckwheat concentrate reduces serum glucose in streptozotocin-diabetic rats. *Journal of Agricultural and Food Chemistry, 51*, 7287–7291.

Kirtikar, K. R., & Basu, B. D. (1993). *Indian medicinal plants*. Dehradun: International Book Publisher.

Kumar, D., & Kumar, S. (2008). Phytochemical investigation and antioxidant activity of Chenopodium album. *International Journal of Plant Sciences, 3*(1), 166–167.

Lozano, I. (2001). The therapeutic use of Cannabis sativa (L.) in Arabic medicine. *Journal of Cannabis Therapeutics, 1*(1), 63–70.

Malinowsky, B. (1944). *A scientific theory of culture and other essays*. Chapel Hill: University of Carolina.

Pandey, A., & Bhatnaga, S. P. (2009).Antioxidant and phenolic content of the bark of Artocarpus lakoocha. *The Pharma Review*, 173–176.

Prakash, P., & Gupta, N. (2005). Therapeutic uses of Tulsi with a note on Eugenol and its pharmacological actions: A short review. *Indian Journal of Physiology and Pharmacology, 49*(2), 125–131.

Richards, A. I. (1939). *Land, labor and diet in Northern Rhodesia*. London: Oxford University Press.

Shah, P. P., & Mello, P. M. D (2004). A review of medicinal uses and pharmacological effects of Menthapiperita. *Natural Product Radiance, 3*(4), 214–221.

Singh, P., & Singh, A. (2012). Evaluation of latex extract of euphorbia royleana for its Piscicidal and Muricidal activities. *World Journal of Agricultural Sciences, 8*(5), 520–524.

Spiller, G. A. (2001). Dietary fibre in prevention and treatment of disease In G. A. Spiller (Eds.). *CRC handbook of dietary fibre in human nutrition*, Washington: CRC Press LLC.

Tomotake, H., Liu, Z., Huang, X., Ishikawa, W., Kayashita, J., & Kato, N. (2001). Feeding buckwheat protein suppresses 1, 2-Dimethylhydrazine-induced colon carcinogenesis in rats. In *Proceedings of the 9th* International Symposium *on* Buckwheat *at Chunchon*, pp. 595–601.

Upadhyay, V., Kambhoja, S., & Harshaleena, K. (2010a). Antifungal activity and preliminary phytochemical analysis of Stem Bark Extracts of Juglans regia Linn. *IJPBA, 1*, 442–447.

Upadhyay, V., Kambhoja, S., Harshaleena, K., & Dhruva, K. (2010b). Anthelmintic activity of the stem bark of Juglans regia Linn. *Research Journal of Pharmaceutical Phytochemistry, 2*, 465–467.

Chapter 4
Mystic Healers

> *...When someone gets healed, the Kingdom of God is revealed, for His Kingdom is a Kingdom or wholeness, of well-being, and of life...*
>
> Billy Joe Daugherty

Abstract Communities have diverse sensitivities regarding the cause of diseases and these impersonations took years to develop and still prevail in the region. People believe that evil spirits are the root cause of large number of human sufferings which often appear in the form of diseases and these beliefs still prevails in society irrespective of caste and class. Curing through spiritual means, states that ailment can be cured by holy trust together with appeal and/or sacraments that inflame a divine having the power to remedying illness. Viewed as extremely sanctified, with height as a persistent commemoration to the eminence of human soul and its vastness, Himalayas exemplify universality of human realization. Communities living in Himalayas call mystic healers not only for seeking opinion for social problems but for getting refuge from illness caused by supernatural entities. Mystic healers act as priests, social workers, friends and advisors, psychologists, psychiatrists and philanthropist to traditional Himalayan communities and they seek refuge in the transcendent realm of supernatural world.

Keywords Magico-religious healing · Mystic healers · Mediators · Witchcraft · Exorcism · Spirit possession · Sorcerer · Shamans · Evil-spirit · Evil-eye · Magico-religious practices

Communities have diverse perceptions regarding the cause of diseases and these impressions took years to develop and still prevail in the region. Apart from minor diseases, a number of diseases are considered to occur due to imbalance of body humours. The cold climatic conditions are believed to be the cause of headache, fever, cough, respiratory diseases, body aches, etc. Of the various assumptions made to find the reason, some of possible causes of diseases are impact of supernatural powers, evil-spirit, evil-eye, ancestral wrath, magic and planetary influences.

Disease is taken to be more serious if it manifests itself in the form of pain, loss of appetite, and any imminent life threatening symptoms. The onset of serious disease makes stresses people and the solution to such problems is always sought

P. Gupta et al., *Healing Traditions of the Northwestern Himalayas*,
SpringerBriefs in Environmental Science, DOI: 10.1007/978-81-322-1925-5_4,

in the celestial metaphysical world. People believe that not paying due gratitude and reverence to local deities', makes them annoyed and their wrath results in disease. In such situation, people seek the help of mystic healers. An attempt is made to cure the disease by making use of magico-religious techniques. These can invoke the divine power which intervenes in handling the cause of disease. According to tribal communities living in Kinnaur and Lahaul and Spiti, faith healing provides gradual relief from pain; at times, brings about a sudden relief, and people use it in place of, or simultaneously with, other healing methods.

The very idea that the curse of folk deity causes diseases has given them the recognition providing remedy of diseases. Worship of village Gods is an essential part of life of rural people, especially during the local village festivals and after crop harvest. There are demonic deities, feminine deities, serpent Gods, saints, whistling spirits and other mystic and sacred benign forms which are revered as Gods and Goddesses. People believe that Gods and other divinities meditate on mountain peaks and legendary heaven and metaphysical world is located in the midst of Himalayas. While conversing with people, it was noticed that in some areas, certain days of the year and specific sites are marked to make special offerings to these deities.

People in some parts of the state make offerings to the Goddess 'Shetala' for protection against eye related problems as also to prevent the attack of smallpox or chickenpox. People narrated-

> Every year, the first Tuesday of March is marked for the worship of Goddess 'Shetala'. The child after recovering from chickenpox is taken to the temple of the Goddess to seek the blessings in future.

There is a temple of 'Brahmani Mata' in Tarapur village near Palampur, which is visited by people from all over state. A local person narrated:

> Some years back, a resident of the village suffered from smallpox. He could not be getting relief. One day his grandmother had a vision, in which the Goddess instructed her about a hidden idol buried at a particular spot. Goddess directed her to install the idol in a temple otherwise the village will have to suffer the consequences of epidemic. The villagers installed the idol in the temple and the patient was cured. Till date the offerings are made to the Goddess.

'Shanti Nag', who is believed to be the incarnation of Shesh Nag, is visited by people for cure from smallpox. The temple is situated in district Mandi. Likewise, Shikari Devi, in district *Mandi* is visited by patients suffering from epilepsy. Churdhar, a famous shrine in district Sirmour is visited by people for getting treatment of incurable diseases. Goddess 'Naina devi' in district Bilaspur is visited by thousands for being blessed with good eyesight. People believe in the role of magical performances in inducing diseases. To cure any physical or psychological ailment, people seek the help of mystic healers. People visit 'Mahunag devta', whose temple is located in district Mandi, for getting cured from mental problems. Besides this, there is a temple of 'Bhooteshwar' in Karsog, which is visited by many. According to people:

> The temple of 'Bhooteshwar' has five-faced idol of Lord Shiva and behind the idol of Lord *Shiva* there is the idol of *Mahakaal*, which is usually kept veiled. People believe that if anyone looks at it, he or she will die. Even the priest, while performing worship tries not to face the idol.

Karsog valley is also believed to have numerous spirits- both evil and good. The 'Kali Tamsheera', for example, frightens the shepherds and the cattle in the jungle. The 'Yogmarg devta' is believed to eliminate ghosts and is considered to be the incarnation of Hanuman. The 'Battad devta' is responsible for rodent infestation in the house, 'Putna' causes harm and illness in small children and the 'Dhoomri jhoor' is believed to control storm and rain. The 'Narsing devta' is considered the incarnation of Lord Vishnu and is worshipped in all households. The 'Veer Jogni' is worshipped by magicians and so is the *Mahakaal*.

There are few village deities which are visited for the treatment of mental problems. Some of these include 'Nagdhamuni devta', village Balahan, Mandi district, 'Shirgul devta', village Shantha, district Shimla, devta 'Bendra', village Deem, Kotkhai tehsil, 'Shalnu' and 'Mahasu' devta, village Brara, tehsil Rohru, 'Kaleshwer devta', village Kotighat, Kumarsein tehsil and Goddess 'Bhimakali', village Deoti-Khoundu, district Shimla. Not only this, there are few sites, where deities such as 'Lakhdatta' and 'Pir' resides and are thronged by people. These deities are believed to be of Islamic origin and are frequently visited for getting rid of skin diseases. People visit these sites on Thursday and offer a broom, soap and mustard oil. 'Baba Dudhiya Than' in district Kangra is visited by patients of snakebite. People have deep rooted faith and they believe that even if the snake-bite victim is able to reach the place, the problem is surely cured. 'Baba Shibbo Than' in district Kangra is also visited for the same purpose. According to legend:

> Baba 'Shibo' is the incarnation of Lord Shiva. He was completely handicapped from birth, but he kept himself involved in the worship of God. He mediated on 'Gugga', a saint, who blessed him with a boon. He was blessed to be a spiritual healer of snake-bite. He was positioned high and his clan was blessed with the power to heal the poison sufferer by serving only drinking water thrice in a day. Even the dust of place where he meditated has the curative properties, for which, it is taken away by the people

In addition to this, 'Gugga' is believed to be the Snake God and is the protector deity. The patients of snake-bite are treated with hymns and herbal formulations and the deity is propitiated by offering baked bread and incense.

The shrine of 'Baba Balak Nath' located on the boundary of district Bilaspur and Hamirpur is visited by childless couples for begetting a child and removal of spirit possession. Each pleading visitor is given holy ash drawn from sacrificial fire which burns continually. The same is also used by the priests in rituals for removing evil-spirit. At times, auspicated rice or wheat grains, mustard seeds are given to the patient for the purpose.

In Kinnaur, Hindu Gods and Goddesses are honoured and people seek their help in getting rid of their problems. The 'Koti devi' temple is visited both by Hindus and Buddhists. The temple's architecture has influence of both Hindu and Buddhist art. 'Narayans' and 'Nag' are worshipped in Kinnaur. 'Narayans' are low-ranked, while Nags are linked with fertility and prosperity. In addition to this, village deity play a very important role in the life of people and every village has its own village deity with a temple dedicated to it. These Gods are brought out from their temples in palanquins on festive occasions. A committee constituted by the village deity supervises the temples of village gods. The committee consists of president, oracles popularly known as *Grockhs, Shumats, Pujari* or priests, Secretary, and cashier or *khajanchi*, *Chalia,* who lift palanquins and *bajgisaa* or the musicians. The village deity is not a statue but an authority, who behaves like common human beings with sentiments and sense of pride. The institution of village Gods is not a matter of chance. There has been legend behind each one of the Gods and this practice has its roots in the midst of ancient past. The oracle is the interpreter of deity, and narrates the power, miracles and curses inflicted by the deity. When charged with the power of the deity, the oracle shakes his head and starts uttering words which gives an impression as if the deity itself is conversing. The words uttered by the oracle are accepted by the devotees as the prophecy or order of the benign form of deity. These village Gods direct social customs and the people cannot afford to disobey deity at any cost. Thus, deity is not only considered the main ruler of the activities but also as the symbol of village culture. Village deities worshiped in some of the villages of district Kinnaur includes, 'Thakur Devta', 'Devi Mathi', Chhitkul; 'Devta Thakur' and 'Vishnu Narayan', Kalpa; 'Bhimakali' at Kamru; 'Devta Markaring', Khwangi; 'Devta Shishering', Pangi; 'Devta Nag', Sangla and Sapni; 'Devta Parogang', Bhabha; Devta 'Kumshu', Kafnu; 'Devi Usha', Nichar, 'Devta Nag', Natpa, 'Devta Milakyum', Akpa; 'Dvevta Dabla', Chango and Pooh and 'Devi Durga', 'Devta Kasurajas' and 'Devta Guruka' in Ribba. A local native of village Lippa narrated:

> Lord Tegatshu Narayan' is thronged by people who suffer from wrath of evil spirits or magical powers. The deity is prayed for getting the solutions of the problem. After the consultation, a day is fixed by the committee with the approval of deity for removing the magical spell. Victims are directed to bring required material and milk. On the fixed day everyone assemble in the premises of the temple and the oracle calls them one by one. The sufferer is made to sit before the deity and is covered with a sacred cloth of deity. The oracle communicates with the deity and using a locally available thorny plant, tries to ward-off the spirit and finally the offerings are made to the deity.

In Pattan valley of Lahaul, a special festival is organized to drive away the evil-spirits. During the festival the priest moves within the village with a burning stick in his hand, meant to drive away the evil-spirits. Besides pleading to folk deities for cure or prevention from illness, a number of natural water bodies are known for their curative value. Hot water springs of Tattapani, Manikaran and Markand are known for curing skin diseases. In Manali, hot sulphur springs have been tapped and created as Vashisth baths where people take bath. People believe that the water act as antiseptic and the salts in water cures insect bite heals wounds and abrasions.

People have great faith in the healing powers of Vashisth baths. Hot water spring of Thopan in Kinnaur is also visited for the same purpose. If the phenomenon has to be explained scientifically, warm baths in the normal course, relieve aching muscles and arthritic joints. Warm water promotes the blood circulation which is always beneficial in hastening the body's natural healing processes. People have experienced the effects of sulphur dissolved in hot springs which does promotes healing. Water of streams for instance, *Devnalla* near Sangla and *Rukti khud* near Rajgarh in district Sirmour is known to be effective in the respiratory problems. In the recent years, there is discussion on the decline of hot springs; for instance, the hot springs of Tattapani are going to submerge with the advent of Kol Dam. This will not only have the impact of the surrounding ecology, but once lost will no longer be made available to the patients, who use to visit these. Water of *Kunal Pathri,* a place in district Kangra, is considered effective in the treatment of various ailments. The water is collected by people, who come from far off places. A waterfall near Vashista village, district Kullu is visited by people for performing certain rituals concerned with small children, with a belief that doing so at that place saves the child from wrath of evil-spirits. Worship of 'Khwaja peer' in villages of Bilaspur is very common. The deity is believed to control rainfall and related activities. Water of tank at Johrji, district Solan, is believed to have curative properties and is frequently visited for the same.

In some areas, it is believed that if a woman has no children it may be due to the interference made by evil-spirit. In such case, the woman is taken to a holy place where she undertakes ritualistic performances. She is made to creep in through a narrow hole in a big stone and on coming out bathe after leaving one garment at the spot. This frees the woman from the evil influence. Sundays in the months of January–February and August-September are considered auspicious for this ceremony. Dip in *Acchara Kund*, sacred water pond in district Kangra, by a childless lady proves to be useful. *Rukmani Khud* in *Tarer* village of Bilaspur is visited by barren ladies for getting a child. Some localities narrated that if a barren lady bathes in the pond and tie her hair ribbon with the grass grown in the premises, is surely blessed with a child.

Local Goddess, 'Simsa'in Kangra is visited by childless women with a hope of getting a child. During their visit to the temple, the women continuously pray and spend few nights in the temple premises, where they are made to sleep and during the dream, the Goddess appear and give them a fruit or any other object. The type of object given by the Goddess helps in predicting the future. If the Goddess blesses with a fruit, it signifies a child, if it is rope and sickle, it indicates that the woman has to work hard throughout her life and she will not be blessed with a child. Here the object visualized in the dream helps in predicting the likelihood of getting the blessing of Goddess in form of a child. Similarly 'Hurang Narayan' of village Hurang in district Mandi is visited by issueless couples for begetting a child. 'Bijli Mahadev' temple in Kullu is visited on occasion of annual ceremonies during which the followers carry a chariot of the deity and invoke his blessing for bringing rain and good crop. 'Bijli Mahadev' is also believed to help in worldly affairs and birth of a son. 'Kailoo', a famous deity of Chamba, is worshipped during the pregnancy. The expectant mothers visit the temple for the safety of the embryo and secure delivery. After the birth of child, the deity is worshipped with a piece of cloth and ear of sheep. A sheep is reared in the name of deity and offered to the deity with a piece of cloth sprinkled with blood of sheep.

Goddess 'Brijeshwari' and 'Chamunda' in district Kangra are visited by people from all over the state and even outside state for seeking her blessings. Both the Goddesses are worshiped by the people who are mastering in magical practices. Lohari festival is celebrated in Brijeshwari temple, which continues for 7 days. According to a legend:

> Goddess 'Chandika' killed demons and took rest in Kangra on the night of Lohari festival. During the fight with demons, the Goddess got some injuries and her devotees applied clarified butter as ointment on the wounds. At that time Kangra was known for herbal treatments. In the memory of the occasion, people even today, celebrate festival is the same manner

People smear butter on the statue of Goddess. The ceremony is known as *Gritmardhan.* The butter is removed after 7 days and is distributed among devotees and is believed to cure various diseases.

4.1 Mediators Between Materialistic and Metaphysical Worlds

People living in Himachal Himalayas believe that evil spirits are the root cause of large number of human sufferings which often appear in the form of diseases and these beliefs still prevails in society irrespective of caste and class. There are number of ways by which these sprits afflict people. One such thought which exists among people implies, that these spirits inhabit deserted places and attack people thereby resulting in creating troubles which often manifests in the form of disease. This is referred to as *chaya padana* or *parchawa padana*, i.e. infliction by shadow of evil-spirit. In this, the evil spirit enters the body of a person and makes him sick and as a result the person starts behaving abnormally and if not treated for a long time, condition gets worse. Evil-eye is believed to be another cause of illness especially among children. As a result of this, children develop sudden disease and fall sick without any explainable reason. In some cases, it was narrated that the condition of the patient became so serious that the victim even thought of committing suicide rather than suffering with the inflicted disease.

Witchcraft, common in the state, is learned or acquired through extensive training and consistent practice. Women learn this art and once they acquire it, they start using it on people and harm them. The witch is commonly known as *dagnis*. Certain days are marked for practicing witchcraft. One such day comes in the months of August–September, is commonly known as *dagyali* or *dagchaudasi*, a night before no moon night. On such occasions the witches perform various magical acts in the cremation ground, evoke evil spirits and make them attack enemies or even other people. This sometimes results in death of the victim. People consider these days as bad and they try to stay indoors especially during nights. Also, they do not accept sweets from anyone on these days. Besides these days', no moon night or full moon night of any month and Tuesday, Saturday and Thursday are other days which are considered optimum for practicing witchcraft. A resident of village Bagain, in Shimla district narrated:

> Since the month of August is thought to be unlucky, hence no celebration takes place in this month. It is believed that in this month, all the Gods, Goddesses and Local Deities leave earth for a meeting in heaven and the evil spirits get activated. Hence, for the whole month the folk musicians visit from one village to another and beat drums after sunset to awaken the divine powers and ask for their protection. For this, they are given food grains by the villagers. In this month, worship of local deities is performed and oil lamps are lit daily. People in this area believe in the unseen powers and existence of evil spirits. Linked with this belief, there is one festival which is celebrated in our area and is known as *Dagvansh*. This comes on the 14th day of no moon night. The day is believed to be of witches who gather and practice witchcraft. In order to protect themselves, every household prepare *chausari,* an ethnic food, cut it into pieces at the entrance of house and throw its pieces in all directions

A similar type of belief exists in the district Kinnaur. People believe that during winters, the village deities visit heaven. The farewell and welcome occasions are celebrated with great pomp and show. People anxiously wait for the return of deities. On coming back they foretell the future of villagers. In the absence of deity people try to keep themselves indoor, especially during evenings because of the fear that evil-spirits haunt the place in absence of presiding deity. People hang a locally available thorny plant at their doorstep to prevent the entries of spirits.

Opra or magical charms are induced by enemy or some relative to physically or mentally harm a person. *Mooth*, another deadly form of magic and cross road motifs are some other paranormal methods which are used in disease transference. The two are practiced at such a place which can serve as most vulnerable for the victim. The practitioners chant demonic verses and perform magic rituals followed by throwing of magical stuff in the air. This if happen to come in contact with victim, results in the death or serious illness of victim. The cross road motif is usually conducted at cross roads where four roads from different directions meet. In this, the magical charms are laid on seven different types of grains tied in black or red cloth along with earthen lamp, dry coconut, mustard seeds and kept at crossroads. If anyone happens to touch or cross charmed items, becomes the victim and results in transference of disease.

In some parts of district Sirmour and district Shimla, there is a popular belief that the practitioners of magic make their victim unhealthy and finally results in slow death. Herein, food to be given to the victim is offered to the local deity with a prayer to save the family from any health problem and for the purpose victim's sacrifice is made to the deity. At times, even the thought of harming the victim may induce illness and death. This is popularly known as *vish dena* or magical poisoning. Sometimes whole family gets affected by bad luck, ill-health and suffering. The power of harming others in thought has been gained and mastered over a period of time. Attack of evil spirit is believed to be the cause of this. In some cases the magical charms are implanted or buried under the house, which often manifests itself in form of disease or death of family member. In yet another method, the magic-practitioners or witches, who are able to perceive the evil spirits or souls; catch hold of spirits and make them enter a person or house and cause nuisance which, often results in disease and restlessness.

Exorcism is method of driving out the evil-spirits from a person or place which they are believed to have possessed. Exorcism is ancient technique and is the part of the belief system of many communities including the Himalayan communities. There are different categories of folk healers dealing with supernatural world. They have acquired the skill or power from some expert trainer or ancestors to commune with mystical world. In local dialect, these people are called by different names as *dau*, *chela* or *maali*. These are mainly the oracles who undergo trances and establish contact with deity or supernatural powers. Patients don't have to reveal their history, symptoms and nature of problem to them. Being associated with village deity, they are easily accessible and use prayers as method of treatment, besides, using incantation, holy water, holy ash, grains or incense.

In debates pertaining to spirit possession, scholars have used numerous terms such as spiritualism, spiritism and spirit medium spiritualism. However, the most common term is generally used in two senses:

- To describe a metaphysical theory that asserts the reality of a non-material, spiritual world- a view common to many religions; and
- To identify a system of beliefs and practices with the objective of communicating with the supposed spirits of those who have died.

Spiritism is a belief linked likelihood of conversing with the spirits of the departed or the dead and the practice of attempting such communication, usually with the help of a medium who is believed to act as an intermediate with the spiritual world. The conjurer possesses skills to establish communication with spirits of departed soul for finding the reasons for body ailments. Belief in the possibility of communication with the other world is an ancient technique and common among mountain communities. It has been held by people but widely alienated by era, space and culture. However, it has lost its grip in the western countries after the psychiatrists began to draw attention to the subconscious powers of human psyche. Most important aspect of spiritism is spiritual healing. The conjurer records the signs and nature of trouble is not required to be revealed by patient. The cause of distress is enquired from the demised souls. Contact is established with demised soul whose help is sought in resolving conflict or disagreement. They only recommend solution which helps in revelation of misfortune and related illness. These skills are confined to certain clans hence these are not easily available. Conjurer is believed to be 'inspired' or 'possessed'. He usually speaks in a voice not of his own, and acts in a manner alien to his normal nature, uttering prophesies and display knowledge which has been acquired as ancestral gift.

The Sorcerer on the other hand, is skilled in performing magical acts, including suffusing or elimination of evil-spirits. Symptoms and nature of problem are examined by them both at physical and meta-physical level. Reason is explored by examining the patient and appearance of symptoms. They make use of magical spells, amulets, threads etc. for minimizing the effects of magic. They can eliminate or suffuse malevolent spirit in victim. Basic means of exorcism are *mantras* and *yajnas* derived from Tantric traditions. The method followed by practitioners of exorcism in Himachal includes the use of *mantras*, and religious material, signs, images, amulets, etc. The exorcist invokes God or other souls to intervene with the exorcism.

In case of attack of any evil spirit or magic, people visit exorcists and even seek the help of local deities. Folk deities have their own priest or Shamans who are generally known as *Gurs*. They are the mediators between the world of spirits and the world of men. They have the ability to converse with the spirits and thus help in solving problems of people. The system of shamanism involves a range of traditional beliefs and practices concerned with contact or interaction with the spirit world. Himalayan people believe that spirits play important roles in human lives and there are people who can control and /or communicate with the spirits for the benefit of societies. Shamans use diverse processes and techniques, as chanting of verses, *yajana*, etc. to evoke spirit and after establishing a communication, find out the cause and remedy for the problem. They even possess the power of calling the spirits and make them enter any body. Thus, they can treat illnesses or sickness because of their ability to diagnose and cure suffering. Shamans have been credited with the ability to know and control the supernatural world. By using their power, they control spirits and force them to follow their command. At times, the exorcists may act as snake or insect bite healers, herbalists or even bone-settlers. The treatment is generally done before the deities or at times the deities are invited at home. The worship takes place on fixed days of the week or month. Patients reach the deities on the fixed day and before the treatment process starts, patients are called one by one and Shaman listens to their problems. During the process, the Shaman communicates with the spirits and answers the queries of the patients on behalf of the invoked deity or divine spirit. At times, these Shamans become aggressive and even beat the patient with special sacred chains. But, it is believed that beating does not hurt the patient but hurts the evil spirit present in the body of the patient. During the visits to different tribal areas, a few shamans were seen in the possessed state:

> In a village nearly 45 kms from Reckongpeo, a Shaman named X, people and the priest of local deity, gathered in the courtyard of a temple. Shaman locally called *Grockhs*, was strongly built and was of medium height. He in his twenties, with fair complexion, wearing traditional attire, behaved normally in non-possessed state. Nothing in his behaviour distinguished him from other tribal folk of his age and class in the non-possessed state. He seemed to be well-mannered, articulate, intelligent and active. But, after attaining the possession, there was a dramatic physical change, while standing, he staggered, appears to lose his balance, begun to sway and it appeared that he may fall onto the bystanders. Soon the entire body started vibrating, at times, it turned rigid. He was seen lurching back and forth from toe to heel, the intensity of which increased with the passage

> of time. Soon he started emitting sounds and groans. Changes in eye and posture were noticeable and at climax, he picked up shackles to ward-off the evil-spirit. Once the possession state was attained, the speech, gestures and mannerism changed. Amidst drumming, singing, he started delivering his message or advice and prescribed remedial measures. At times, he behaved benevolently, greet individuals and extend suggestions. This off course required the undiverted attention of entire audience. One among the public having ability to commune with shaman, interpreted his commands.

At times, goat or sheep is also slaughtered during the possession ceremony to appease the deity. Until the deity gets appeased, the process continues and when the spirit confesses and asks for forgiveness, possession starts ceasing. The cessation of activity is accompanied by slow quivering which indicates that the possession will soon come to an end. It was found that the depth, involvement, loss of control, strength of behavioural changes is not constant during the possession. The shamans have control over their body and keep conscious against any injury to their own body or the other's.

The possessed state is attained to prescribe a treatment, diagnosis of severe maladies or misfortunes, and even failure of crops, trade or any other enterprise, barrenness or childlessness. There is fixed time for all ritualistic performances which is decided by the deity and drumming is integral part of invocation. It creates an atmosphere in which the possession becomes expected. The shamans also interpret the dreams and visions. There are various causes of possession and one among these is that it is required by the deity to perform the useful tasks such as healing and annihilation of evil-spirit. If the cause of possession is deity, who requires the service of shaman, the necessary training is given to him so as to prepare him for useful service of community and deity. The shamans and priests through both observation and divination offer advice on etiology and disease descriptions. In addition, they are capable of elaborating the ideas of heredity and patient's responsibility as causes of certain illnesses, make prognosis and prescribe right treatment. The experienced priest is quite familiar with the symptoms which suggest that the patient suffers from acute mental problem. Within his cultural assumptive world, the spiritually possessed shaman is capable of diagnosing and treating physical and mental ailments. The shaman is also able to tell which disease, he can cure or not and advice accordingly to opt for the advice of another experienced healer. Even if one opts for another treatment, the healing by shaman still remains operative. Hence, the physical and spiritual treatment goes on simultaneously.

Possession ceremonials can add to social solidarity and stability by providing communal public opportunities with supernatural sanctions to people with anti-social behaviour, especially linked with witchcraft practices. It also helps a person to get rid of feeling of weakness and loss in the midst of disorder. Thus, possession can be seen as individual therapy, group therapy, but, both prophylactic and curative. On one hand, it adds to the aesthetic interest of people and on the other hand drumming, gatherings, etc. are both social and ceremonial. The phenomenon of possession reaffirms the possibility of communication with supernatural world.

Among the psychological phenomenon, important one is clairvoyance or perceptions of things beyond human senses or intelligence; xenoglossy, in which the person who acts as medium, speaks or writes in a language unknown to him and cryptesthesia, which is the ability to make contact with persons, places or other objects of unknown origin, that the medium is fully able to describe. As far as the existence of these phenomena is concerned, the folk healers residing in the North-western Himalayas do possess these qualities and they have evolved their own mechanism of communication and making predictions. They are able to commune with the supernatural agencies and convey their message to the victim, which in some cases is understood and interpreted by special spokesmen who are attached to oracles or shamans. The individuals do possess extraordinary powers, the nature and limits of which are beyond human intrusion and understanding. However, this requires the fusion of moral forces, constituted by values; psychic forces conditioned and imposed by nature and religious forces offered by divine munificence.

At times, the charmed amulets are given to the patient, to tie around the arm and neck along with some holy ash or grains. The holy ash is to be smeared on the forehead whereas the grains are meant for consumption. It is believed that the amulets cure the disease and offer protection against the attack of other spirit. In case, the amulet fails to treat the patient then treatment is done by ritualistic performances, including *yajana* and making animal sacrifice. This is usually conducted at mid-night. The patient has to perform the *yajana*. Certain special *yajanas* are performed only at specific times and are believed to have magical impact. A tribal narrated that a woman was not conceiving and when she was brought to exorcist, the attack of evil spirit was detected as the cause of problem. During the treatment, the woman vomited red threads, nails and hair. According to the exorcist, her relatives made her suffer. Treatment of disease caused due to the magical act or *opra*, involves the use of amulets or inhalation of sacred incense. To remove the effect of poison, the exorcist is invited to perform rituals. The deity is evoked, who spots the place where magical charms are buried. The magical charms usually consist of bones, vermilion, ash, nails, hairs etc. The evoked deity removes the charms and offers the protection. In some cases, to drive away the evil-spirit the exorcist, by using special magical rituals caught hold of spirit and pinned it down. During the process the iron nails are used to pin down the spirit.

In case of treatment of children affected by the attack of evil-eye, *Capsicum annum*, *Swertia chirayita* household garbage and broom stick are moved over the head of the child and burnt in fire. Burning of dried *Asparagus adscendens* also cures evil-eye. Animal body parts are used for driving away evil-spirit and protecting against evil-eye. Bear hair is burnt and its ash is used for removing the effect of evil-eye. Owl bone or its ash or its meat is used for treating diseases caused due to the effect of evil-eye.

Jhadha, the simplest form of exorcism, is mainly done for the treatment of bite of venomous animals, evil-eye and even for physical and mental sickness. During this, patient is made to sit before the healer who tries to drive away the evil-spirit or disease by chanting *mantras* and or using plant twigs of *Vitex negundo*, brooms, peacock feathers, holy ash, mud, etc. The healers don't disclose the healing techniques to anyone because of popular belief that its effect is reduced if disclosed to undeserving. To drive out the spirit, plant twigs or broom or feathers are moved from head downwards or swirled around the head in circular fashion. Various physical ailments cured by *jhadha* include headache, herpes, skin-diseases, body pains, jaundice, mumps, tonsils, earaches, etc. Some communities have received the art of healing as God's gift while some others have inherited it from ancestors. In case of jaundice, the *jhadha* is done by using plant twig of *Vitex negundo, which is moved over the head of patient and touched with mustard oil,* the latter turns yellow after it thereby signifying that disease has been removed. *Jhadha* is also done in case of insect or snake bite. This not only removes the poison but cures the shock and after effects of the insect or snake bite.

For treating evil-eye by *jhadha*, the same is done by making use of peacock feather. A number of other methods are also used for getting rid of evil-eye. These include the application of *kajal*[1] on forehead and eyes, use of black thread, amulet, etc. Wheat bread is baked from one side and after moving over the head of victim, is thrown away or kept at crossroads. In some areas, a handful of common salt is swirled over the head of child and thrown in running water. For treating mumps, three *Capsicum annuum* fruits, three *Sapindus mukorossi* fruits, *Hordeum vulgare* grains, iron nail and a copper coin are moved over the head of the child and kept on crossroads.

People in Kinnaur district also believe in spirits and this has shaped and influenced the belief system of tribal community. One can see the horns of animals hung at the entrance of every house which is believed to ward-off the evil-spirits and at the same time brings good luck to the house.

Ancestral adoration is quite common among people in Himachal Pradesh and people believe that if the same is not done suitably, a curse in the form of illness may befall the family. It is also referred to as *pitri dosh* or *'pitri khot'*. In case of diseases caused due to ancestral wrath, direction is given by priests to make offerings to the ancestors in the form of special feasts for Brahmins. In addition, there is conjure, who has attained the ability to communicate with the departed soul. Their help is sought to know the exact cause of misfortune or disease. The concept of deeds conducted in the earlier births, which is the basis of philosophy of *karma*, also persists among mountain communities. People regard good health, either as blessings of God or the result of good deeds done in the past. They believe in *paap* (sin) and *punya* (good deeds) and accept that disease is the result of sins committed in previous births. In case of disease due to bad deeds, treatment is prescribed by the priests/astrologers, which generally involve organizing of special spiritualistic performances to satisfy the planets and stars. For reducing the effects of certain planetary influences, some charitable acts are also prescribed. Worship of some Gods and Goddesses and trees is recommended by the astrologers for reducing the adverse effect of planets. Lighting of an oil lamp at crossroad

---

1 *Kajal* is the kohl used as a cosmetic by women.

or under sacred tree, placing of seven grains at crossroads is suggested for lessening the planetary effects. People follow these methods with a belief that by doing so, the effect of disease is abridged.

4.2 Sacred Healing by Buddhist Monks

Although Bön is practiced in district Kinnaur but Hinduism and Buddhism are also followed in the district. These three, along with traditional shamanistic practices have shaped the religious milieu of the region. In lower Kinnaur, there is more impact of Hinduism, whereas in Mid-Kinnaur there is prevalence of mixed religion, i.e. Hinduism and Buddhism, while in upper Kinnaur there is more influence of Buddhism. People in mid-Kinnaur worship both Hindu and Buddhist deities. 'Dabla' is one of the main folk deities, which is worshiped in entire district. Mount 'Kinnaur Kailash' is considered as the sacred mountain and is thronged by people. Buddhist monks or popularly known as lamas, play a significant role in the life of people. They are invited for conducting religious ceremonies, from birth to death. People send their children for practicing monkshood or Lamaism. They are made to learn Tibetan scriptures which not only help them in attaining spiritual knowledge but also acquaint them with mystical ways of healing. One can find stones slabs with prayers engraved on them at the entrance of almost every village and on enquiring people it was found that the prayers were written on them by Buddhist monks at the time of natural calamities or epidemics and placed on the boundaries of the village to provide protection against the attack of misfortunes. These are frequently visited and worshiped by the villagers. Buddhism is based on Buddha's tenet that:

> Suffering is unnecessary, like a disease, once we really face the fact that suffering exists, we can look more deeply and discover its cause; and when we discover that the cause is dependent on certain conditions, we can explore the possibility of removing those conditions

During an interaction with a Buddhist monk, the spiritual aspects of healing in Buddhism were explored. According to Buddhist monk Lord Buddha has taught various ways of healing which people have preserved, refined over the centuries and have passed down to following generations. Buddhism, believe in spiritual and psychological aspects which are associated with suffering and often affect the body. There are different ways which can be used for spiritual awakening of body, removing bondages and relaxation of body. He further substantiated that they perform special ritualistic performances for the benefit of individuals who are ill or deceased.

One can observe old women meditating in tribal villages of Kinnaur and Lahaul and Spiti, using prayer wheels, prayer flags hanging around bridges and houses. The traditional prayer wheel is a small device which is used for spreading divine vibrations and blessings. The prayer wheel consists of roll of paper imprinted with verses, and is kept around an axle in a cylindrical container. The same is spun round and round. People believe that spinning of prayer wheel make an appeal to lord 'Chenrezig', who is compassionate and take care of everyone. Even the touching and turning of wheel results in purification of body and most people keep this wheel in their houses. All these are the ways of pleasing God, asking for well-being of community.

People have an old tradition of printing prayers on colored flags and hanging them across mountain passes, over houses and places of worship, bridges or anywhere where the prayers may meet the wind. This helps in spreading the essence of prayers to the entire world and appeases the power of divine spirits thereby fulfilling the wishes of the person who hung them. Prayer flags create an ambiance of peace and hope wherever they are flown and invoke feelings of kindness, harmony, wisdom and strength in addition to protection against dangers and evil. People pray for the happiness of entire universe, for the removal of sufferings of everyone and ultimately liberation of all. According to people, prayer flags give peace, happiness, and health for oneself, for ones loved ones and neighbors, for strangers in the area, and even for ones enemies. *"Om Mani Padme Hum"*, is the well-known verse of 'Chenrezig', and all teachings of Lord Buddha are contained in it. Chanting of this verse makes an appeal to the lord for his kind consideration. Even if one views its written form, it has similar effect. Chanting of divine verses is one of the most primitive healing techniques, which invokes the Medicine Buddha who blesses medicines and produces healing effects. There are mantras which are dedicated for healing specific illnesses or for longevity, removing problems of life, purification of food and so on.

Most ritualistic performances involve the burning of incenses. Incense is prepared according to traditional method using natural ingredients such as flowers, leaves, grass, wood, bark, spices, and aromatic herbs found at high altitudes. Different types of incense are prepared based on ancient medical texts. The purpose of using incenses is to purify the surroundings, relaxation, meditation and as an offering to God. These relieve stress and tension, purify the air and are beneficial for body aches. These help in achieving calmness relive headaches, rheumatism, gout, allergy, gastric and urinary problems. These sharpen the senses, and improve concentration. Some may act as insect repellent, some have soft cooling refreshing effect and removes tension and sleeplessness. Important ingredients of these incenses are myrrh, musk, sandal wood powder, saffron, spruce, juniper, rhododendron, cinnamon, holy basil, cardamom, cloves, nutmeg, camphor, jasmine and other medicinal and aromatic ingredients. These ingredients have their own affect, for instance, e.g. myrrh, is used in tantric initiations, Juniper clears, stimulate, and strengthen the nerves and so on.

4.3 Plants in Magico-Religious Rituals

The *Vedas, Puranas, Upanishads* and other ancient scriptures contain a detailed account of trees, plants, wildlife and their significance in the life of people. *Yajnavalkya Smriti*[2] mentions cutting of trees as an offence whereas *Kautilya's Arthashastra*[3] mentions the necessity of forest management and expresses the concern for all living creatures. Even in Islam, one finds a close harmony between ecology and man. The *Vedic* literature has scientific and religious description of nature. The place of plants and trees in ecology had been well understood by people, which is evident from the great epics and mythological books. The great epics like *Ramayana* and *Mahabharata* contains numerous incidences where God's relationship with nature has been described.

Rural communities have evolved a number of folk proverbs where they have linked the human behaviour and attitudes with the peculiarities of plants or animals. This indicates that people are well aware of the unique characters of these and have learnt this over a period of time, for instance, tree of *Butea monosperma* or *flame of the forest* is widely distributed in lower Himachal, and is used for timber, resin, fodder, medicine, and dye. It is associated with spring season, and finds mention in folk literature especially in poems and songs where the bright color of plant is linked to orange flame of fire. The morphological characteristic of this plant is that it always has three leaves. In folk literature this peculiarity of plant is linked with human who is just the same whether in comfort or adversity and in local dialect it is said that-*Bashkal kitnai bashau plah-de chauni pach,* means "it does not matter whether there is a heavy monsoon or a light one, the tree of *Butea monosperma* always has not more than three leaves."

In another proverb the fertility of women is linked with the flowering of *Crocus sativus* plant. The plant is barren; its flowers fail to produce viable seeds-thus its reproduction is carried out artificially, which is a bit difficult. Thus, its fertility is compared with that of infertile women. Here the proverb depicts the knowledge of people regarding the flowering of *Crocus sativus* and its link with the life itself where it used to show impossibility in a childless mother. In local language it is said, *Aj niputi kal niputi, Kesar fulti sadda niputi,* which means today and tomorrow she is without a son, she is without a son even when the saffron blooms.

People have linked the character of plants with human behaviour. The plants with fragrance and beauty are considered good and so is the human behaviour; whereas the thorny plant is always considered troublesome. It is said, *Chdmbe mule, Bhekhlai jammi,* means, under a fragrant tree, there grew a thorny plant. This proverb is used when a well-to-do man has an ignorant son. Here one finds the observational abilities and analogical wisdom of rural communities regarding the

---

[2] *Yajnavalkya Smriti* is the "well written" and "most homogeneous" text of the *Dharmaśāstra* tradition. It reflects a level of complexity in comparison to many of other texts of its time. It was written by Sage *Yajnavalkya* during the Gupta dynasty.

[3] *Kautilya's Arthashastra* is a book concerning economics written by the great scholar *Kautilya.*

environment they live in. Folk herbalists are the repository of traditional knowledge especially on the utilization of plants for medicinal purposes. They pass on the knowledge to the next generation through small couplets, for instance, *Jeethi, Bhnah, Basuti, Barna Tethi Manhu Keinha Marna*, means, a man cannot die of disease in an area where *Vitex negundo* (bhana), *Adhatoda vasica* (basuti) and *Acorus calamus* (barna) are found, provided he is aware of the method of using them. This proverb not only speaks of the value of these plants but at the same time because of a rhythm which sets in allows one to remember the names of these plants. The words *barna* and *marna* sets a rhythm in the couplet. Another verse says- *Para, Gandhak, Vish, Dhatura, Hartal, Suhaaga, Tank-Tank Bhar Pura Pipal Jeerea Dohno Lejeeje Bhukhar Bahan Pakar Bahar Keejae,* meaning, by using *para*, *ghandhak*, *vish*, *dhatura*, *hartal* and *suhaaga* along with *pipali* and *zeera,* one can always turn out fever. The words *lejeeje* and *keejae* sets a rhythm and make everyone aware of the seven ingredients used in treatment of fever. Numerous stories and legends are linked with plants which talk about the important characteristic feature of plant. A popular story from *Kinnaur* revolves around the plant '*Shel*'. '*Shel*" is a medicinal plant which grows in the *Bhaba Pargana*, whence many kinds of medicinal plants are said to be obtained. The subsequent story is told about it:-

> Once upon a time a shepherd was grazing his flock on the meadows of "Shel Samang" (Shel: medicine, and Samang: the meadow of herbs), when he beheld a dead snake lying on the ground. After a while another snake came to the very spot where the dead snake was lying, and seeing his companion dead, he immediately took a leaf of a particular herb, put it to its mouth and instantly restored him to life to the astonishment of the shepherd, who had secretly witnessed the whole scene and had recognized the life-giving herb. After playing there for a time, both the snakes went away. Then the shepherd came down to the place, killed one of his sheep and put a leaf of the herb to its mouth. The sheep at once got up as one awakes from sleep. The shepherd was overjoyed to find such an herb, and made many experiments with it successfully. One day he even beheaded one of his friends and restored him to life. Then he told his companion to put him to death and restore him to life with the herb, which he pointed out to him. His companion killed him, but, unfortunately forgot the herb, so that he could not bring him to life again.

This folk legend on one hand mentions the antidote property of the "*shel*" plant and on the other hand gives a message that overexploitation leads to devastation. If one tries to exploit nature, the nature takes its revenge and rendered helpless in servicing human requirements. The shepherd kept experimenting with the plant but ultimately died because of ignorance of his friend. The friend forgot the herb because of lack of knowledge and was the cause of his friend's death.

Plants occupy a prominent place in the life of Himalayan people. The mythological beliefs still prevail in the Himalayan society. It is believed that a person is honoured in heaven for 1,000 years if he resides in a house where the holy basil is grown. Plants, besides being the part of natural resources, have a magico-religious role to play.

It was found that many plants are considered sacred and are often protected, worshiped and sacrifices are made to gratify these. Offerings are placed under these plants. *Ficus religiosa* trees grown in villages are worshiped and underneath these, magico-religious rituals are performed. Tree of *Ficus bengalensis* is also considered sacred. During religious and social ceremonies, these trees are worshipped and offerings are made. This shows that people still believe in mystical, religious and social importance of plants in their culture. *Ficus bengalensis* is usually associated with fertility and prosperity and is worshiped by women for the long life of husband and even by childless women for getting a child. *Ocimum sanctum* is worshiped by womenfolk throughout the year. The plant is not only considered sacred but it is also used for various medicinal purposes. Bark and leaves of *Zanthoxylum armatum* are believed to expel evil-spirits. *Calotropis gigantea* is used in magico-religious performances for the treatment of diseases caused due to planetary influence. *Vitex negundo* is considered holy and used in healing treatments, especially those involving sorcery. It is used in exorcism. Some plants are considered sacred because of their close association with a deity, for instance, tree of *Aegle marmelos* is linked with Lord *Shiva*, *Ocimum sanctum* with Lord *Krishna* etc. Leaves and flowers of *Thevetia nerifolia* are used for worshipping lord *Shiva*. Leaves and fruits of *Aegle marmelos* are also used for worshipping lord *Shiva*. Its fruit, flowers and leaves are all sacred to *Shiva*, liberation's summit. Planting *Aegle marmelos* trees around home or temple is as sanctifying, as worshiping the deity with its leaves and water. *Withania somnifera* is used for *tantric* initiation. *Betula utilis* is used for the preparation of amulets and the tree bark is used for writing religious manuscripts.

Plants are used during sacrificial fires to achieve the desired physical, psychological and spiritual benefits. On burning, various chemical changes take place. During the sacrificial fires, a number of substances are used, which are offered in the fire. These consist of *samidhá,* i.e. wood, and *havan sámagri,* i.e. mixture of aromatic herbs. Wood to be burnt is dried and made free from dust, insects and worms. It is cut into small pieces of varying sizes called *samidhas*. The wood of sandal, cedar, mango, sacred fig, banyan, etc. is used for the purpose.

The mixture of aromatic herbs is prepared with an appropriate combination of odoriferous substances, sweetening agents, substances with healing properties and medicinal herbs. The main odoriferous substances include saffron, musk, agar, sandalwood powder, cardamom, nutmeg and camphor. Substances with healing properties consist of ghee, milk, dry fruits, sesame seeds, and cereals like wheat, rice and barley. Sweetening substances consisting of sugar, dried dates, resin, honey, etc., and medicinal herbs such as *Tinospora cordifolia, Bacopa monnieri, Convolvulus pluricaulis, Mesua ferrea, Terminalia bellirica, Terminalia chebula,* etc. are used for the purpose. Different combinations of these herbs are used for the treatment of specific diseases through *yajana*-therapy. The *yajana* not only purifies the environment but removes the foul odors, bacteria and insects. Scientific studies have shown that the partial oxidation of hydrocarbons and decomposition of complex organic substances produce formaldehyde, which is a powerful antiseptic and has germicidal action. Insects are killed or driven away when they come in contact with volatile oils like camphor, which are diffused in the environment during the performance of *yajana*. The aromatic substances get diffused in the air after *yajana* and offer protection to life against harmful organisms. Some other

Table 4.1 Plants used in Magico-religious Practices

Sr. No.	Name of the plant(s)	Magico-religious significance of plant
1.	*Abutilon indicum*	Used for detoxifying the effects of poisoning during religious ceremonies
2.	*Achyranthes aspera*	Used in *yajana* and *tantric* practices to ward-off the evil-spirits and lessening the effect of magic. Its seeds are used in *yajana* to please Goddess *Durga*. It is used for making amulets and its seeds are boiled and consumed by saints living in forests. Used for treating snake bite
3.	*Aegle marmelos*	Leaves, fruit and flowers are all sacred to *Shiva*, liberation's summit. Planting its trees around home is as sanctifying, as worshiping the deity with its leaves and water. Dried leaves, fruits and stem are used in *yajana*, which imparts longevity
4.	*Asparagus racemosus*	The whole plant along with roots is worshipped during the marriage and other religious ceremonies. It is worshipped as the form of lineage deity. Used for hypnotizing in *tantric* rituals
5.	*Azadirachta indica*	Dried leaves are used for removing evil spirit
6.	*Bambusa sp.*	Its wood is used in various religious ceremonies and performance of certain rites such as death rites
7.	*Bauhinia vahlii*	It is considered pure hence used for religious purposes for making leaf plates
8.	*Berberis lycium*	Its stem and dried roots are used in *yajana* to please Goddess 'Baglamukhi'
9.	*Betula utilis*	Tree bark is used in the preparation of amulets and writing sacred manuscripts
10.	*Brassica juncea*	Used in *yajana* performed to ward-off evil spirits. It is also believed to please Goddess 'Aasuri Durga.
11.	*Butea monosperma*	The flowers are offered to Goddess Kali and its wood is used in *yajana*
12.	*Calotropis gigantea*	Plant is used during the ritualistic performances for the treatment of diseases caused due to planetary influence. The plant is worshiped and mustard oil is poured over it. The plant is also used for worshipping lord *Shiva*. Dried stem of plant is used in *yajana* for appeasing Sun God. The dried stems dipped in clarified butter are used for the purpose
13.	*Canarium resiniferum*	Used for *tantric* purpose
14.	*Cannabis sativa*	Leaves are used to worship lord Shiva
15.	*Capsicum annuum*	Used in various magico-religious practices mainly to drive away evil-spirits
16.	*Citrus medica*	Used in magico-religious ceremonies and tantric practices, especially for making sacrifices
17.	*Cocos nucifera*	Used in religious ceremonies and tantric practices, for making offerings and sacrifices
18.	*Colocasia sp.*	Leaves are used to drive away evil spirit

(continued)

Table 4.1 (continued)

Sr. No.	Name of the plant(s)	Magico-religious significance of plant
19.	*Coriandrum sativum*	Used for magico-religious purpose
20.	*Corydalis govaniana*	The plant is used in for removing evil-spirits
21.	*Cucurbita sp.*	Used in *tantric* practices, especially for making sacrifices
22.	*Cyperus scariosus*	The plant is directly related to Goddess 'Kali'. It is used in *yajana* performed for bad dreams and nightmares
23.	*Datura metel*	Its leaves, stem, leaves and flowers are offered to lord Shiva
24.	*Eclipta alba*	Used to drive away evil spirits and *tantric* practices
25.	*Fagopyrum esculentum*	Used in religious ceremonies by people in Kinnaur. Its flour is consumed during the fasts
26.	*Ficus bengalensis*	Leaves used in religious ceremonies. The tree symbolizes the Trinity of Lord Vishnu, Brahma, and Shiva. The tree is worshipped by childless couples
27.	*Ficus religiosa*	Its leaves are used for various religious ceremonies. It is one of the five sacred leaves used in religious ceremonies. It is believed that Lord *Brahma* resides in the tree trunk. It is worshipped on Saturdays to reduce the planetary influences
28.	*Girardinia palmata*	The plant twigs are used to ward-off evil-spirits. It is believed that if any amulet is kept in its leaves, no impurity can ever affect it
29.	*Grewia oppositifolia*	The ropes prepared from its stem fibres are used in religious purposes, as preparing of garlands, etc.
30.	*Juglans regia*	Fruits are used in various religious ceremonies. The fruit is worshipped on the occasion
31.	*Juniperus sp.*	For making incense
32.	*Jurinea dolomiaea*	Plant is used for preparing incense for religious purpose
33.	*Mangifera indica*	Leaves used for religious purpose as one of the five sacred leaves. Leaves are used for preparing garlands and stem is used in *yajana*
34.	*Musa paradisiaca*	The fruit is offered to deity during religious worship. The trunk of tree is erected during the religious and social ceremonies at entrances, as they are believed to be auspicious
35.	*Nelumbo nucifera*	Flower is used for worshipping Goddess 'Lakshmi'. The plant is linked with prosperity. Its seeds are used in *yajana*
36.	*Nerium indicum*	The leaves and flowers of plant are used for worshiping lord *Shiva*
37.	*Ocimum sanctum*	Considered as most sacred plants in Hindu religion and planted in most households. The plant is believed to sanctify and guide to heaven, all those who grow and worship it. Leaves are also given to a person at the time of death
38.	*Oryza sativa*	Rice grains are associated with Goddess 'Lakshmi' and are believed to be a symbol of prosperity. There are numerous festivals connected with the sowing, planting and harvesting of rice. Rice mixed with turmeric is popularly used in religious rituals

(continued)

Table 4.1 (continued)

Sr. No.	Name of the plant(s)	Magico-religious significance of plant
39.	*Pandanus odorifer*	Essence of flower commonly known as "*Kewda iter*" is one of the most popular perfumes extracted and used in India since ancient times in religious ceremonies. Its extract is used for flavouring various foods, sweets syrups and soft drinks
40.	*Piper nigrum*	Used in Tantra and tantrik rituals
41.	*Poa cynosuroides*	The plant has a great religious significance. It is believed to be highly pure and is used in birth, death and marriage ceremonies. During the solar or lunar eclipse, the dried plant is put in containers containing eatables because of the popular belief that it protects the same from the effect of eclipse. It is used in certain religious ceremonies, especially those performed in connection with ancestors.The plant is plucked by priests on a special day often called "*Kusahpattani Amavasaya*". This grass is then dried and tied in small bunches and distributed to the people. Grass is also used to prepare small mats used during worshipping
42.	*Prinsepia utilis*	Shrub is considered auspicious and worshipped. Oil of its seeds is used for various religious purposes
43.	*Prunus cerasoides*	Leaves of plant are used in religious ceremonies especially in worshipping Lord Shiva. Its wood is considered sacred and is used in *yajana*
44.	*Rhododendron sp.*	Used in religious ceremonies, especially by the Buddhist people in Kinnaur. Its garlands are used to decorate the temples of village deity
45.	*Sapindus mukorossi*	Used in magico-religious procedures mainly for the decreasing the effect of evil-eye
46.	*Saraca asoca*	The tree finds mention in Vedic literature including epic *Ramayana*, where it was worshipped by Goddess Sita. Its worship is considered beneficial for removing sorrows and sufferings
47.	*Saussurea obvallata*	Flower is used for worshiping, especially by people in Kinnaur
48.	*Spondias pinnata*	It is one of the five sacred leaves used for religious purpose
49.	*Terminalia arjuna*	It is believed to be the tree of 'Swati', a lunar mansion and in *Yajana*
50.	*Thevetia neriifolia*	Its leaves and flowers are used for worshipping lord *Shiva* on the occasion of Mahashivratri
51.	*Trachyspermum ammi*	Seeds are used for warding-off evil-eye. For the purpose, the charmed seeds are burnt and the victim is made to inhale its smoke
52.	*Triticum aestivum*	Seeds and flour used in various magico-religious purposes. Seeds are used to get rid of planetary influences
53.	*Vernonia cinerea*	It is an extremely rare herb mostly used in Tantric practices
54.	*Vigna radiata*	Seeds are used in various magico-religious and tantric practices. The seeds are donated to priests, especially on Saturday, for reducing the effect of planetary influences

(continued)

Table 4.1 (continued)

Sr. No.	Name of the plant(s)	Magico-religious significance of plant
55.	*Vitex negundo*	Twigs used in magico-religious performances especially to ward-off evil-spirits
56.	*Zanthoxylum armatum*	Used to ward-off evil-spirits
57.	*Zea mays*	Cobs are used for worshiping water God. Its seeds are used in religious rituals and form a part of seven sacred grains

Plants used for *Yajana*

*Cedrus deodara, Aquilaria agallocha, Terminalia belerica, Cassia fistula, Rosa sp., Ficus racemosa, Holarrhena antidysenterica,*Myristica fragrans, *Nardostachys grandiflora, Curcuma zedoaria, Mucuna pruriens, Acacia catechu, Sesamum indicum, Convolvulus pluricaulis, Crocus sativus, Emblica officinalis, Mesua ferrea*

Plants used in magico-religious practices

Cynodon dactylon, Acorus calamus, Elettaria cardamomum, Calendula officinalis, Terminalia chebula, Tinospora cordifolia, Curcuma longa, Hordeum vulgare, Syzygium aromaticum, Piper betle, Adhatoda vasica, *Withania somnifera, Emblica officinalis, Brassica juncea, Areca catechu*

plants are considered sacred because these shelter objects of worship like a deity. In some villages, *Bir* and other folk deities are believed to reside in the bushes; and people consider such patch of land as sacred and worship it. A number of plants or their parts are used in magico-religious ceremonies (Table 4.1).

Thus, plants serve a variety of cultural and symbolic functions and are linked with cultural heritage of Himalayan communities. They not only play a role in the cultural life of people, but are also central to magico-religious ceremonies. The folk stories, legends and proverbs linked with plants not only depict the traditional wisdom of people, but also speak about the deep ecological concern which people have for nature and its components. The wisdom must be preserved and passed on to the coming generations.

While noticing the roles of folk healers, it was found that besides playing the role of healer, they act as priests, social workers, friends and advisors, psychologists, psychiatrists and philanthropist to traditional Himalayan communities. Supplicants come to them from surrounding areas as well as from far-off places. Possession endows them with the power of authoritative utterance, for which they claim no personal responsibility. Their view and judgments are supported by public opinion. They weigh, sum-up and clarify the personal problems of victim with authority. The cult of local deity is thought to be beneficial to the communities and their commands and judgments are acceptable to everyone irrespective of caste, creed or social status. Folk healers thus, focus and support the hopes and aspirations of entire community, besides offering protection and security from evil forces.

Chapter 5
Traditional Herbalists

> *...Every simple plant remedy is blessed and gifted by God and its Handmaiden nature to such an extent, that according to its own nature and way, it has the power to heal, strengthen, allay pain, cool, warm up, purge, and sweat...*
>
> Heironymus Bock, Kreuterbuch

Abstract North-Western Himalayas are the treasure house of medicinal plants. For several generations, the local inhabitants have been collecting plants to use them as medicine. The plant gatherers have different sets of techniques for herb extraction. In case of disease, the people, visit traditional herbalists, who examine the patient and make diagnosis. They are capable of treating a variety of disorders. Herbalists usually prescribe medicines which are in the form of powders, decoctions, medicated oils, creams and ointments. They claim that the information they possess, has been passed on to them as a part of the family traditions. The healers are capable of treating the common ailments, and some even specialize in certain areas ranging from pediatric medicine to orthopedic medicine and from snake bite to traditional birth attendant. The traditional medical system has persisted in the region for a very long time, its healing significance and what is retainable of this system and how these can be upgraded through education, licensing and incorporation into state health planning still needs to be linked.

Keywords Folk herbalists · Indigenous mountain communities · Herbal formulations · Infusions · Decoctions · Concoctions · Traditional therapeutic procedures · Pediatric medicine · Indigenous dermatology · Traditional orthopedic practitioners · Traditional birth attendants · Amchis

Pharmacognosy is the study of remedial measures which are obtained from nature and herbal medicine or "herbalism" is also the investigative research which looks into the therapeutic properties of herbs. For instance, the bark of willow tree is believed to contain large amount of salicylic acid, and has been used for millennia as an effective pain reliever and fever reducer. Research studies carried out around the world have shown that plants are capable of synthesizing a wide variety of chemical compounds that can perform vital biological functions. Many of such phyto-chemicals have useful effects on long-term health, and can be used to

P. Gupta et al., *Healing Traditions of the Northwestern Himalayas*,
SpringerBriefs in Environmental Science, DOI: 10.1007/978-81-322-1925-5_5,

successfully cure human ailments. Phyto-chemicals intervene in human body through processes alike that of chemical compounds of contemporary drugs; thus herbal medicines do not differ from conventional drugs in terms of their action. This allows herbal medicines to be as effectual as conventional medicines. The use of plants as medicine is as old as human history itself and the Ethnobotany is believed to have paved the way for modern medicine. The term "Ethnobotany" was coined by John Harshberger in the year 1896. According to him, Ethnobotany is the study of plants used by primitive and indigenous communities. Since then, it has been defined as the long-established wisdom of ethnic communities regarding the adjoining floral diversity and the study on the usage of plants by the individuals of a particular culture. According to Hamilton, ethno-botany is:

> …the study of how the people of a particular culture and region make use of indigenous plants," while the ethno-botanist explores how plants are used as food, shelter, medicine, and clothing, for hunting, and in religious ceremonies. It is the science studying "the relationship between a given society and its environment and in particular the plant world…

It has a significant role in conserving nature and culture. Traditional knowledge systems being nascent are not only linked with the knowledge of plants as medicine and food but also with the sustainable utilization of resources. In the year 2001, scientists identified 122 compounds which are used in contemporary medicine and were known to be derived from "ethno-medical" plant sources and 80 % of these have had an ethno-medical use identical or related to the present use of active Phyto-chemicals. The use of herbs to treat ailments is common among all societies, and is often more reasonable than buying costly modern drugs. The World Health Organization (WHO) estimates that 80 % of people in Asian and African countries presently rely on herbal medicine for primary health care. Many of the herbs and spices used to season food also produce useful medicinal compounds.

5.1 Dependence of Indigenous Mountain Communities on Forests

The North-Western Himalayas are widely known treasure house of medicinal plants. Himachal Pradesh, one of the northern states of India, spreading over 55,673 km^2, is located in the North-Western Himalayas. The Forests of the state are known for their splendor which add feather to the Himalayan crown. Except for small valleys, whole of the state is mountainous and is bestowed with diversified forests comprising of rich floral and faunal wealth. Forest land in Himachal covers an area of 37,033 km^2 (Table 5.1) and constitutes about 66.52 % of total geographical area of the state. Area under tree cover is 14,668 km^2; whereas area

Table 5.1 Geographical distribution of forest in Himachal Pradesh

#	Area Km^2	Percentage of geographical area	Percentage of forest area
1. Geographical area	55,673	100.00	–
2. Forest area (legally classified)	37,033	66.52	100.00
3. Area under tree cover	14,668	26.35	39.61
4. Very dense forest	3,224	5.79	8.71
5. Moderate dense forest	6,383	11.47	17.24
6. Open forest	5,061	9.09	13.66

Source FSI Report 2009, H. P. Forest Department

under dense forests is 6,383 km^2. However, when compared to other Himalayan states the forest cover in Himachal Pradesh is comparatively low. In addition to timber, the forests are rich in medicinal herbs, fodder, grazing plants, fiber, gum, resins, wild fruits, etc. and the State Forest Department issue permits for collection of non-timber forest products. Some of the medicinal and aromatic plants having special significance are found only in the state. Of the twelve districts of Himachal, maximum forest cover (48 %) is reported from district *Sirmour* and lowest from district *Lahaul and Spiti* (1.3 %). The state contributes 2.12 % to the total forest cover of the country. Twenty different types of vegetation have been identified from the state. These includes, Alpine meadow, Alpine scrub, Rhododendron, Chilgoza, Chir pine, Blue pine, Deodar, Dry deciduous, Ephedra, Hippophae, Juniper, Mixed conifer, Moist deciduous, Oak, Riverine, Sal, Scrub, Temperate broadleaved, Temperate grassland, Temperate scrub and Non-forest. Based on the available information, the flora of Himachal Pradesh consists of about 180 families comprising about 1,038 genera and about 3,400 species. Asteraceae with more than 328 species is the largest family followed by Poaceae and Fabaceae. *Carex* is the most dominant genera (48 species) followed by Polygonum (37 species) and Poa (33 species). Hence, the rich floral diversity of the state not only supports the livelihood of its inhabitants but also provides wide opportunities for the researchers to work on the biodiversity. Medicinal plant diversity in the state is spread across more than 100 plant families with the highest represented families being Asteraceae, Rosaceae, Ranunculaceae and Fabaceae.

'People–nature' interface in the state is seen along with a variety of livelihoods. The ecological niche and livelihood strategy, which are essential components of subsistence livelihoods, remained reliant on customs or traditions but increasingly became immaterial with the passage of time. From the times of yore, local communities inhabiting the Himalayas had dependence on natural resources, especially forests, which varied from settled pastoralism dependent on local pastures and fodder resources to nomadic pastoralism to high meadows. The forests, besides providing land for extension of agriculture activities, have been exploited for fuel wood and leafy bio-mass for compost. Prior to state's take-over of forests for systematic supervision, forests were largely under the control of local communities.

5.2 Herb Collection and Processing

For several generations, the local people in the North-Western Himalayas have been collecting medicinal plants. The purpose of collection was to use them as medicine. Earlier these were used in conventional health care systems and presently they are again in demand because of shifting of people towards naturopathy. This has resulted in the steady development of herbal market. Methods of identifying herbs, knowledge of collection and usage pattern have passed on from generation to generation. In some areas, the entire family is involved in herb collection. People specifically go to the pastures and collect medicinal herbs. The elder generation train the younger ones regarding the identification of plants, their use, time and method of collection, etc. Collection of medicinal plants by folk herbalists depends on several factors as:

- Nature of plant part to be used, i.e. dried or fresh;
- Part of plant to be utilized i.e. root, stem, leaf, flower, latex, gum, resin, fruit or seeds;
- Season of collection;
- Time of collection;
- Site and Method opted for collection;
- Form in which the plants are required for preparing formulation; and
- Quality and quantity required or desired for preparing formulation.

5.3 Methods and Collection Time

The plant gatherers have different sets of techniques for herb extraction, for instance, herbs growing in the environs of farmlands and in surrounding forests are collected by men, women and children along with their other tasks like fuel and fodder collection or grazing. The grazing of cattle is generally combined with the extraction activity. The collection of medicinal plants from pastures and distant forests is undertaken by men having adequate knowledge on collection tactics. Those gathered from high altitudes include *Dactylorhiza hatagirea, Ephedra gerardiana, Nardostachys jatamansi, Saussurea costus, Aconitum heterophyllum, Picrorhiza kurrooa, Podophyllum hexandrum, Swertia chirata, Valeriana jatamansi, Rauwolfia serpentine.* Local herbalists or *Vaidyas* have adequate knowledge and they not only visit the surrounding areas but also move to far-off places. Those who have inherited the knowledge of healing from their forefathers often know the place of collection, collection time, identification and method of extraction. As far as collection from distant places is concerned, the gatherers leave in groups with their bags and cover long distances. Some plants which are not available in the region, but are required for formulation are purchased from local vendors. The local people also collect some medicinal plants and sell them to herbalists or local merchant.

The herbs so collected are dried and processed for further use. At times, the gatherers also gather plants of religious or cultural importance along with the medicinal plants. The seasonal collection patterns vary considerably, but remain confined between the months of March and November. At times, competition for resources results in premature extraction which is often very destructive. The professional herbalists having proper knowledge disclosed that following aspects are taken into account while collecting a medicinal plant:

Day, time and season: The herbalists are well aware of day, time and season of extracting medicinal plants. Some sacred plants with medicinal value are harvested on specific days and specific time. For instance, cutting of *Ficus religiosa* is prohibited on Sundays; similarly leaves of *Ocimum sanctum* are not plucked on Sunday and Tuesday. Some old healers even narrated that special prayers are made before picking the plants. *Poa cynosuroides*, a sacred grass is collected only once in a year and that too on specific day. Most herbalists disclose that they worship plant and pray before them. In this way, they recognize the spiritual and curative powers of plants. They believe that by doing so the potency of the plant increases spiritually.

Identification: The folk herbalists are adept in recognition and segregation of plants. At times, identical plants or plants of same genus but different species growing in vicinity have different attributes. One may have medicinal properties whereas the other might be poisonous. But, the age old experience of these healers help them in making clear-cut identification of plants.

Part to be collected: The healers have understanding of collecting specific part of plant and its importance as a medicine. They knew when, how and to what extent the part of the plant has to be extracted.

Collection of bark: The bark of a tree collected for medicinal purposes is cut at specific place from the trunk so as to retain its curative properties. This method not only checks the damage of plant but also ensures that the bark can be collected again in future. Here the herbalists take into consideration the age of plant and also its state i.e. fresh or dry.

Collection of roots: While gathering roots of medicinal plants, herbalists take into account that after extracting the required amount, the remaining part is not injured and plant survives.

Collection of leaves, buds and flowers: Leaves, buds and flowers to be used in formulations are picked up at specific time. The healers are precisely familiar with the flowering time of each plant, they make use of. Hence, they visit the field at that particular time and gather the required parts. Care is taken to leave behind some representatives of collected species so as to prevent them from extinction.

Collection of fruits and seeds: Collection of fruits is done by hand picking or gathering of fallen fruits from ground. The status of fruit, whether ripened or raw is taken care of before gathering them as per the requirement. Mature seeds are collected and dried for medicinal purposes.

Collection of whole plant: In case the whole plant is required, the collector generally takes out the entire plant from the earth along with underground parts, but care is taken not to damage the surrounding plants. The seasonal collection pattern of different medicinal plants varies from region to region.

5.4 Collection Strategies

The extraction season for most of the medicinal plants starts in the month of March. The collection of different species in different areas continues for three to 4 months. There is strong competition for collecting medicinal plants among the gatherers during the extraction season. Gatherers often divide the forest areas among themselves for exploration. Most of the medicinal plants are perishable hence the collection is done on demand. Plants which can fetch good market price, i.e., have good commercial value are sold in the market but also kept for household purpose which are used either as food or in home remedies. Collection of herbs depends on its accessibility. If the herb is scarce, the traders don't buy them hence the gatherers gather such herbs only for personal use.

5.5 Processing of Medicinal Plants

Before selling the herbs, these are required to undergo primary level processing, which varies from species to species. Drying, segregation, cleaning, grading and slicing/cutting are the most common processes performed by the gatherers.

Sun Drying: It is a low cost technique which protects the plants from fast degenerating. The collectors go for sun-drying of plants to reduce the moisture content of medicinal plants. Some of the plants do not require direct sunlight for drying. Hence, such plants are dried in shade to retain their effectiveness. On an average 6–7 days are required for drying medicinal plants.

Segregation: In the next step, collectors segregate the herbs, where the marketable part is separated and grading is done. Cleaning and sorting is done according to the size and quality of dried plants, grading is done in accordance with the size, quality and quantity.

Marketing: The gatherers sell their collection to local agents or shopkeepers. Extraction of medicinal herbs by villagers is an age old practice in the state which is undertaken largely by almost entire family however, the degree of dependence on medicinal plants for monetary benefits varies. The activities associated with extraction, processing and trading of medicinal plants are not merely seasonal, but are also related to a range of uncertainties with respect to availability of medicinal plants as well as their demand in the market.

Procuring Medicinal Plants from other sources: Many plants which are used for preparing medicinal formulations, but are not available locally are procured from local market or brought/ collected from areas. Some of the medicinal plants procured from local market include: *Elettaria cardamomum, Syzygium aromaticum, Piper nigrum, Convolvulus pluricaulis, Cyperus rotundus, Terminalia arjun,* etc.

5.6 Cultivation of Medicinal Plants

As most of the medicinal plants are collected from wild but with increasing demand and decreasing availability, the need for the cultivation of medicinal plants is increasing. It is expected that a vacuum may arise in the supply of raw medicinal plants which are used extensively by pharmaceutical sector as well as by the folk practitioners. This has necessitated the cultivation of medicinal plants which can ensure the availability of raw material to the pharmaceutical sector as well as to the folk herbalists. Cultivation and processing of plants should go hand in hand in rural areas. Systematic cultivation requires precise farming and agronomical requirements which are not only species specific but also depends on soil, water and climatic conditions. Formulation of good agricultural practices which includes proper cultivation techniques, harvesting methods, safe use of fertilizers and pesticides and waste disposal should be encouraged. Research and development work has to be carried out for:

- Optimization of best agronomical conditions
- Organic cultivation
- Selection of fast growing varieties with disease resistance
- Determination of maturity and harvesting time
- Harvesting methods.

In response to WTO regulations, rules have been laid down for streamlining the international trade of medicinal plants collected from the wild. These regulations have not only legalized the collection from the wild but improved the export of cultivated medicinal plants. Cultivation of medicinal plants proves to be highly beneficial. Farming particularly of high value medicinal plants is giving new dimension to the field of agriculture. It can prove a boon for the poor farmers and women having marginal land holding. There are number of benefits of cultivating medicinal plants as:

- Reduces harvesting pressure on rare and slow-growing species which are most vulnerable to threat;
- Guarantees continued supply of raw material;
- Standardization or improvement of genotypes of the cultivated plants can be achieved easily;
- Easy maintenance of quality standards;
- Controlled handling of post-harvest is attainable;
- Production volume and price can be settled;
- Secures stable supply of herbal medicines in the market.

In situ conservation of these resources alone cannot meet demand of folk herbalists, hence there is need to develop cultural practices and propagate these plants in suitable agro-climatic regions. With a view to promote Himachal as pioneer in *'Herbi-culture'*, the state government is motivating farmers to opt for cultivation of medicinal plants on a large scale. The state government has prepared a roadmap for large-scale cultivation of medicinal plants to give thrust to *'Herbiculture'* sector. More than 60 varieties of medicinal plants selected by state government are being cultivated in the state. It is expected that farmers in the state will have a good returns by undertaking cultivation of herbs. According to the roadmap, state's horticulture, forest and *Ayurveda* departments encourage farmers to grow herbs on their own lands, forests and herbal gardens established by department of *Ayurveda*. To give momentum to the cultivation of rare Himalayan herbs, the State is providing technical assistance to the growers and cooperative societies which would cater to the need of pharmaceutical companies manufacturing drugs. The state government is strengthening the agriculture, horticulture, animal husbandry, floriculture and herb cultivation in a planned manner which in turn is increasing the state's economy. Since the state offers favorable climatic conditions for the cultivation of medicinal herbs, herbal gardens are being developed at different climatic zones to inspire farmers to cultivate herbs. Presently, the herbal gardens are located at Jogindernagar in district Mandi, Neri in Hamirpur, Dhumrera in Rohru, and Jungal Thalera. Land holdings unsuitable for traditional farming practices can best be utilized for the cultivation of herbs. The scientists of Chaudhary Sarwan Kumar Himachal Pradesh Krishi Vishvavidyalaya, Palampur and the Parmar University of Horticulture and Forestry, Nauni are working in close association with the farmers to develop economically viable cultivation and utilization of medicinal herbs. Extensive research is being carried out to introduce technological inputs which can enhance the quality and quantity of herbs so that the farmers can fetch remunerative prices for their products. The state is largest supplier of *Chilgoza, Kuth, Dioscoria, Dhoop, Picrorrhiza, Valeriana* and *Ephedera* in the country. New initiatives have been taken to promote herb cultivation through the participation of the masses. *'Jan-Jan Sanjeevani'* and '*Sanjha Van-Sanjivani Van*' campaign, a community driven programme of state government has resulted in massive plantation of medicinal herbs. Every household has been motivated to plant at least one medicinal plant in its premises.

There is a lot of diversity in the medicinal plants and each plant has exclusive characteristics of growth, seasonality, assortment, trade and ethno-botanical importance. Thus, a plant specific approach needs to be adopted for intervention in its ecology and related aspects. Until recently, the unsophisticated methods are used for collection of medicinal plants hence training of plant gatherers is required, which can make them aware of the issues pertaining to extraction, value addition and conservation. Presence of oils, alkaloids or extracts are in their full during a particular season. At that time, the extraction and processing of plant can yield maximum phyto-chemicals; hence the awareness regarding the specific collection schedule and storage needs to be promoted. For adding better value during storage and fetching good prices, plant collectors need to be organized into groups.

5.7 Traditional Methods Employed for Preparing Herbal Formulations

The formulations in traditional system of medicine vary in numerous ways; however the methods involved are highly standardized and take into account the type of plant included and also the problem to be treated. Some of the techniques used by herbalists in preparing herbal formulations are:

- *Kwath*—Infusions (hot teas)
- *Kadha*—Decoctions (boiled teas)
- *Rasa*—(Extracts and alcohols/local wines)
- *Lepa* (Concoctions, creams for external applications)
- *Churan*—(Powdered form of herbs)
- *Vatti*—(Tablet)
- *Dhunni*—(Inhalers/Snuffs).

The competent herbalist is well aware of the conventional methods involved in the preparation of different formulations.

5.7.1 Kwath*: Infusions (Hot Teas)*

Infusions are prepared using the soft herbs, fresh plants with tender leaves and water. Making an infusion is as simple as preparing a cup of tea. For this purpose, the herbalists boil water to which an herb or combination of herbs is added. The boiled water is poured over herbs and allowed to settle/ precipitate for some time. Preparation of infusions is usually carried out in ceramic or earthen pot and according to herbalists the use of metal utensil is avoidable. The ratio of herbs in water or vice versa varies and depends on the remedy. At times, the herbs are chopped-off and at times used in raw form. Similarly, its preparation is done either once in a day and used twice or thrice or at times the fresh infusion is prepared every time it is to be consumed. Infusions are best prepared when required and must be consumed the same day. These can be taken hot, warm, or cold, depending on the type of disease.

5.7.2 Kadha*: Decoctions (Boiled Teas)*

Decoctions make use of more tougher, harder and fibrous plants and their parts such as hard woody stems, barks, dried roots, which need to be boiled to take out the extract. At times, the herbalists soak the dried herbs in water overnight and boil the same for a longer duration, which not only softens the harder material but helps in releasing the active constituents of herbs. The amount of water to be added and duration of boiling depends on the nature of constituents. According to most herbalists, escaping of aroma indicates that the decoction is ready for consumption. The straining is done using a strainer and the herbs are pressed to obtain the best possible extract of boiled herbs. The consumption time, dosage and preparation pattern however varies with the nature of disease. Sometimes the strong decoctions are prepared, where the mixture is boiled for longer duration and the quantity is even reduced to half. Longer boiling time is necessary to soften the larger and harder pieces of herbs. Sometimes the decoctions are prepared in the evening and allowed to settle for the whole night. Stirring of the decoctions is usually done by using the stem of some medicinal plant and herbalists avoid using the metallic stirrer.

5.7.3 **Rasa***: (Extracts, Alcohols, Local Wines)*

At times, the herbalists prefer taking out the extract of plant, especially when the plants possess water insoluble active constituents. These extracts are allowed to ferment and have longer shelf-life. According to herbalists, the older an extract is, the better will be its potency. For preparing the extracts, the herbs are ground fresh or dried and soaked/ boiled in water and allowed to ferment, naturally in the air tight jar, either in the sunlight or in dark, depending on the nature of tincture required. The folk herbalists and tribals of Kinnaur, prepare local wine using apricot, grapes and apples. This wine, with medicinal and curative properties is utilized at household level to get rid of common body ailments, including cough, cold, fever, diarrhea and dyspepsia.

In addition to this, certain macerations are also used by the herbalists and its preparation involves the easiest method. For the purpose, the dried plant material is soaked overnight in water and strained in the morning. The resultant liquid is used for oral application or at times for external application/washing of affected part. This method of preparing formulations is done when the herbs/medicinal plants are too delicate to be heated or boiled and might lose their active constituents.

5.7.4 **Lepa***: (Concoctions, Creams for External Applications)*

Many formulations are recommended for external use only. These includes, *lepa* or poultices which are applied directly on the affected area—normally on boils/ burns, rashes and wounds and as topical pain-relieving medications. These are prepared in number of ways, depending on the type of ailment and mode of applications. Some of these are prepared by grinding fresh herbs in a pestle and mortar and some are prepared by soaking and boiling dried herbs in water and then grinding them to semi-solid pastes. Sometimes, the freshly prepared herbs are tightly pressed to take out the extract, which is applied directly on the affected area. Wet fresh herbs are at times, placed directly on the affected area and tied using the piece of cloth. In some cases, the herbalists recommend the tying of leaves of herbs together with oil or clarified butter.

In addition to this, certain baths and bathing/fomentation remedies are suggested by the folk herbalists. These are usually recommended for external inflammations, skin diseases, body aches, rashes or itching in skin and joint pains. According to the herbalists, the skin is an organ, which is capable of absorbing active herbal constituents or mineral salts dissolved in water. The dermal absorption, through the skin to the underlying subcutaneous tissue, then into the bloodstream, can relieve the pain and inflammations. Besides this, a number of creams, ointments and medicated oils are prepared by using mustard oils, sesame oil, pine oil, apricot oil, clarified butter and bee wax. Some of these are prepared by boiling or heating the herbs in oil/ clarified butter and some by simply soaking the herbs, usually dried, in the oil or clarified butter.

5.7.5 Churan*: (Powder of dried herbs)*

Preparing *Churan,* the powdered form of herbs is the simplest and most commonly used method of preparing herbal formulation. For this, the herbs are dried and grinded using traditional pestle and mortar or stone slabs. The powder can be of single herb or combination of herbs. These are normally recommended with water, curd, buttermilk or cow milk, but the dosage, consumption time and pattern varies with the type of disease. In many cases, the herbalists suggest its intake in an empty stomach and sometimes after meals or in between the meals.

5.7.6 Vatti*: (Tablet)*

The dried herbs, when ground can sometimes be made tablets of. These are small round shaped balls, which are recommended orally with water, yoghurt, buttermilk or milk. The dose and intake occasion and pattern is decided depending on the type of disease. The tablets once prepared are dried in direct sunlight or in shade depending upon the potency of plant and the effect of direct sunlight/heat on its active constituents.

5.7.7 Dhuni*: (Inhalers/Snuffs)*

Many herbalists suggest the use of *Dhuni*, in which the patient is made to inhale smoke or vapors of herbal combinations. These may have medicinal or magico-religious implications on the body. Many of the inhalers have curative effect on lungs and brain and in many cases these relieve the sensory/ nervous systems from pain and stress. In most cases, the herbs are burnt in a close and dark room and the patient is made to sit in it for some time, while in some cases, individual inhalation is also recommended.

5.8 Dosage System

Traditional herbalists use various measuring units and recommend different dosage duration. Local units, for instance, finger length for measuring the size of bark, root, stem, pinch for powdered preparation and numbers for leaves, seeds, fruits, bulbs, rhizomes, flowers and tablespoon for extract of medicinal plants, latex, decoction, number of drops for liquid formulations etc. are used for estimation and fixing the dosage of medicine. The duration of administering the medicinal formulation depends on the degree of sickness. Recovery signs, disappearance of disease symptoms, fading out of disease signs are some of the parameters used to determine the duration of prescription. For instance, some the healers recommend application of two–three drops of oil of *Syzygium aromaticum* for treating toothache. Similarly *Allium sativum* boiled in mustard oil and two drops of preparation are dropped in ear for getting relief from earache. The dosage system also varies from healer to healer but most healers informed that the dose depends on age, physical and mental status of patient. Lack of precision in dosage may at time make the drug inefficient or ineffective.

5.9 Administration of Medicine

As far as the mode of administration of medicine is concerned, it is determined by the nature of ailment i.e. internal or external. Hence the route of administration may be internal i.e. oral and external i.e. rubbing or application of preparation on skin or affected area.

In addition, some healers narrated that for dealing with single problem; medicines can be prepared and applied in different forms. For instance, seeds of *Bauhinia vahlii,* used as tonic can be taken orally whereas root juice of *Bauhinia vahlii* is recommended with buttermilk for treating dysentery. Such accommodating choices enable the patient to select the method of one's suitability. Even the time of application or administration of the drug is determined and subsequently suggested to the patient. It may be early morning before sunrise or late night. The administration of oral formulations may be empty stomach or after meals. Some modes of administration of formulation are linked with the religious aspects. *Vitex negundo* is used for removal of evil spirit or lessening the effect of evil-eye whereas twig of *Zanthoxylum armatum* is kept at doors or windows to avoid the entrance of evil spirits or negative powers.

Placing the root of *Calotropis gigantea* plant in one's pocket is believed to prevent the person from evil-eye or attack of evil-spirit. Even though these magico-religious acts are difficult to be explained scientifically, they are believe to provide psychological assurance to the users. The herbalists also recommend some restrictions which are obligatory when patients are prescribed with some medicine. For example, a patient who takes medicine for dysentery is advised not to consume milk. Consumption of any food item half an hour before and after the administration of medicine is suggested by healers in most of the cases. Intake of rice, potatoes, curd, pickles, whole grain cereals and pulses is restricted for the patients suffering from arthritis.

According to herbalists, the time specification matters a lot in getting good results of medicine. Similarly, a patient getting medicine for treatment of repeated abortions is strictly advised to avoid 'hot' food. Some medicines are prescribed on empty stomach and some after meals, some with hot water and some with cold, some with milk some with curd or buttermilk. For instance, for curing constipation medicine is usually prescribed with hot milk, whereas for curing dysentery, it is prescribed with curd or buttermilk. Thus, the herbalists have devised their own mechanism of preparing and suggesting a formulation depending on the nature of disease.

5.10 Traditional Therapeutic Procedures

Socio-cultural background of any community manages its system of healing and the social-ethos existing within its framework helps in the development of its medicinal traditions. Community's insight which has evolved over the years has not only helped in finding new means of fighting against diseases but have assisted in the survival of old perceptions regarding the diseases and their causative factors. Even today, the rural communities residing in the North-Western Himalayas believe in the role of paranormal in influencing the health and health care systems. Surviving in close association with nature has helped the people in becoming curious for its resource wealth. The beliefs, customs, practices and perceptions with regard to health and diseases are in a continuous process of change and readjustment. Two types of factors affect the health of a community:

(a) **Direct Factors**: Affecting the health of a community directly & governed by traditions, practices, beliefs, ethics, sacred taboos, etc. which helps in spreading or controlling of diseases; and
(b) **Indirect Factors**: Influencing the health of a community indirectly having no connection with spreading or controlling of diseases.

The health of people in Himalayan region is affected by ecological and socio-cultural factors, like climate, topography, remoteness, beliefs and scarcity of resources. Factors directly affecting the health status & occurrence of disease in an individual are settlement pattern and hygiene status; personal cleanliness and food consumption pattern. Factors which affect health indirectly are religion and family's viewpoint on health and health care system opted or practiced

Every culture has its particular rationalization for ill-health. In case of healing rituals, the somatic symptoms are often healed by means of rituals. The distinction between natural and supernatural exists in all cultures. Based on the beliefs of people, the causes of sickness can be due to supernatural entities or by magical means.

Once the disease is diagnosed, the process of treatment starts for which people seek the help of healers. For getting rid of diseases linked with supernatural agencies, evil-spirit, evil-eye, ancestral wrath, etc., people seek the advice of supernatural healers. Use of home remedies is generally the preliminary step in dealing with a disease, but, this again depends on the nature of disease. Home remedies are generally used for small or minor diseases which are of short duration and make use of locally available herbs, roots, leaves, kitchen spices and condiments for curing the diseases.

The home remedies are generally confined to the elders particularly old ladies in the family. Home remedies are generally employed for treating common ailments mainly in children. The household ladies make use of the kitchen condiments and readily available herbs. Mother's milk is used for various medicinal purposes and the breast milk is considered a medicine. The use of mother's milk in case of paediatric medicine is quite common, for instance, the mother's milk is applied on stomach to relieve the stomach-ache. Drops of mother's milk are put in eyes for curing eye problem.

However, when the condition is beyond the control at household level, people visit traditional herbalists, who examine the patient and make diagnosis by simple palpation or feeling the pulse. They claim that the information they possess, has been passed on to them as a part of the family traditions. The healers are capable of treating the common ailments, and some even specialize in certain areas. They are capable of treating a variety of disorders ranging from skin problems, impotency, piles, leucorrhoea, heart related problems, infertility, snake and scorpion bites, mental disorders, arthritis, inflammation, diabetes, jaundice, paralysis, gastrointestinal disorders, diarrhoea, ulcers, kidney stones and asthma to orthopaedic problems. Women have knowledge of birthing and pre-natal and post-natal care. Healers consider plants as sacred and they believe that effectiveness of any herbal medicine depends on the respect and care provided to them and have evolved specific methods of gathering herbs.

Herbalists in the region usually prescribe medicines which are in the form of powders, decoctions, medicated oils, creams and ointments. Though, people go to the folk physicians, they concurrently opt for alternate health care practices. For example, a sick person who is being given prescribed medicine for diarrhoea may also be taken to a folk-healer for evil-eye. Although certain illnesses such as evil-eye are thought to be cured only by sacred healers, this does not rule out the use of herbal medicine to treat the symptoms.

5.11 Pediatric Medicine

Paediatric medicine is mainly practiced at household level. In case of severe problems, help of local herbalists and traditional birth attendants is sought. They are mostly consulted for treating ailments of children such as bronchitis, epilepsy, etc. One of the main components of the paediatric medicine is *Trachyspermum ammi*. This branch of traditional medicine makes maximum use of materials as: mother's milk, *Myristica fragrans, Elettaria cardamomum* and *Syzygium aromaticum*. Mother's diet is especially taken care of if the child is suffering from diarrhoea. For treating diarrhoea in children, *Syzygium aromaticum* is half parched, ground in mother's milk and orally administered to the child. Decoction, given to the child for various digestive disorders is prepared by boiling *Trachyspermum ammi*, *Terminalia chebula* and salt in water. The boiled decoction is filtered, mixed with honey, and orally administered to the child. At times *Acorus calamus* is added to the decoction because of the belief that it helps in the development of brain. For treating constipation in children, decoction of *Cassia fistula* and oilof *Ricinus communis* prepared in milk is orally administered to the child. For treating chest congestion, dry leaves of *Acorus calamus* are ground; the powder is wrapped in cotton cloth and tied around the neck of the child. In this, the powder so tied keeps on sieving out of the cloth and comes in direct contact with chest and relieves the problem.

5.12 Indigenous Dermatology and Cosmetology

'Cosmetology', defined as the study of skin, hair and nails, wherein the emphasis are laid on manicures, pedicures, hair-shaping, occasional hairstyling, shampooing of hair, cosmetic application, body hair removal, hair relaxers, colouring and highlighting of hair and hair extensions or wig treatments. The ancient science of cosmetology is believed to have originated in Egypt and India, but the earliest records of cosmetic substances and their application dates back to Circa 2500 and 1550 B.C, to the Indus valley civilization. The use of cosmetics by women in prehistoric times was as important as it is today, the only difference is that, earlier the cosmetics were prepared using indigenous recipes and unlike present times when synthetic cosmetics are popular. The word 'cosmetic' is used to define substance of diverse origin used to cleanse, allay skin troubles, covering up imperfections and beautify. Inaccessibility of modern cosmetics and inborn urge of looking good, gave rise to efficient domestic remedial measures. For centuries ancient physicians in India practiced the therapeutics of cosmetology and skin disorders. *Charaka Samhita,* a well-known prehistoric therapeutic treatise dealing with basic principles of *Ayurveda,* contains a chapter on the subject. *Atreya Punarvasu* has described eighteen dermatoses and attributed them to the predominance of morbid humorus disturbing the body elements resulting in diseases.

Since times immemorial, people have been using indigenous herbs like, *Swertia chirayita, Emblica officinalis, Terminalia bellirica, Terminalia chebula,* etc. in form of poultices and plant(s)/tree(s) exudates along with cow dung and urine to impart beauty and glow to the skin. Even in the scientific era, due to scarcity of dermatologists in the backward and inaccessible mountainous regions of Himachal, people rely on folk herbalists and faith healers for skin ailments and cosmetological solutions, besides visiting to folk deities for their benevolence.

As far as the dermatological problems are concerned, people living in Himalayan region have developed their own perceptions. According to tribal communities, harsh weather conditions and exposure to cold dry winds are responsible for dry skin and dandruff. Herbalists are of the view that excessive consumption of 'Hot' foods, greasy foodstuff and sweeteners, often causes pimples and acne. According to some elderly women, consumption of molasses or jaggery in summers is the main cause of pimples and acne in the monsoons. The appearance of rashes or reddening of skin, locally known as *baat*, is due to humoral imbalance mainly *pitta*, which symbolizes heat or fire and consumption of food, which aggravates heat, is responsible for this problem.

Besides visiting the local herbalists for seeking help in disease condition, people seek refuge of the metaphysical world. People worship village deities during festive occasions and after each crop harvest, where offerings are made for the welfare of family. Worshipping of Goddess *Shetala* is done every year for protection against smallpox or chickenpox and eye-related problems. Similarly, Goddess *Naina Devi* is thronged by thousands of people for being blessed with good eyesight. People visit shrine of *Lakhdatta* and offer a broom, soap and mustard oil to get rid of skin diseases. Besides praying to local deities for cure of or prevention from diseases, a number of natural water sources are known to be visited for curative capabilities. Hot water sulphur springs of *Tattapani*, *Manikaran* and *Markand* are known for curing various skin diseases. In addition to this, people visit exorcists, who are known to possess the skills of treating various disorders using exorcism tactics which are believed to relieve herpes, skin-diseases, jaundice, mumps, tonsils, earaches, etc. Many families have acquired special healing powers as God's gift and also from the ancestors. Indigenous skin care techniques include the use of naturally-derived ingredients combined with naturally occurring carrier agents and stabilizers, which help in maintaining skin texture. A number of indigenous techniques have been devised to handle dermatological conditions as.

5.12.1 Pimples or **Acne vulgaris**

It is a common human skin disease, characterized by areas of skin with seborrhoea, papules, pustules, nodules and scarring. According to local herbalists, it is caused by the aggravation of heat in the body, which increases due to the intake greasy fried and spicy food, together with stress and tension which results in eruption on

Table 5.2 Powder and tablet(s) suggested for treating acne

1.	Mixture of fruits of *Terminalia chebula,Terminalia bellirica* and Emblica officinalis
2.	*Piper nigrum*, *Piper longum*, *Zingiber officinale* are ground to fine powder.
3.	Dry leaves of *Gentiana kurroo,* leaves of *Azadirachta indica* and seeds of *Piper nigrum* are ground and mixed with molasses to prepare its tablets.
Oils recommended for treating acne	
4.	Chimney smoke, extract of *Cuscuta reflexa* mixed in mustard oil
5.	Mercury, Sulphur and Psoralea corylifolia mixed with mustard oil
Paste(s) recommended for acne	
6.	Roots of *Achyranthes aspera* grinded to fine paste
7.	Paste of roots of *Musa paradisiaca*
8.	Paste of *Euphorbia hirta*
9.	Paste of thorns of *Bombax ceiba* grinded with water
10.	Paste of pulp of *Aloe barbadensis* and *Currcuma longa*

the skin as acne and pimples. A number of formulations consisting of plants and minerals are used for curing pimples, which are either administered orally or applied locally on the affected areas. The main modes of treatments recommended include the use of powder and tablets for oral administration, medicated oils, paste & extracts for local application (Table 5.2).

5.12.2 Scalds, Boils and Burns

Scalds, boils and burns often result while working near fire. A number of formulations, in form of creams, pastes are used for the purpose. The local herbalists recommends the application of extract of *Terminalia chebula, Terminalia bellirica* and *Emblica officinalis,* mustard oil and lime, paste of *Terminalia arjuna* bark, mixture of *Onosma hispidum*, *Tuberosum solanum* and extract of *Cucumis melo* fruit for curing boils. A few herbalists recommend application of paste of *Amebia benthomi* roots for the same. Elderly women folk at household level recommend application of paste of *Lawsonia inermis* for getting relief from burns. They recommend application honey, oil of *Emblica officinalis,* paste of *Tuberosum solanum* or fresh butter as immediate treatment for boils and burns.

5.12.3 Wounds

The cuts and abrasions resulting in wounds often appear accidentally while working in fields or forests. A number of preparations, in the form of extracts or paste, are recommended for local application on affected areas for wound healing.

Some of the commonly used plants are *Cynodon dactylon,Curcuma longa*, *Emblicaofficinalis*, *Azadirachta indica, Dactylorhiza hatagirea* and *Calendula officinalis*. Besides this, use of *fitkari* (alum) was also recommended. Women folk suggest application of paste of *Curcuma longa* rhizome mixed with mustard oil on wounds. While, to combat the inflammation caused by insect bite, herbalists recommend, rubbing of *Cannabis sativa* leaves.

5.12.4 Leucoderma

It is a cutaneous condition, with localized loss of skin pigment, called melanin that may occur after any number of inflammatory skin conditions, burns, intra-lesion steroid injections, post dermal abrasion, etc. The white patches occur all over the body including face, scalp and genitals. According to local herbalists, it is caused by morbidity of liver which results in a deficiency of *pitta* causing poor digestion and building up of toxins in the tissues and is the root cause of this disease. Formulations used for treating leucoderma include the use of oils/pastes which are recommended for local application besides some oral administration. The most commonly used plants and their parts for the purpose were *Psoralea corylifolia, Semecarpus anacardium*, *Cinnamomum camphona, Prunus dulcis* and *Carum copticum.*

5.12.5 Skin Care Cosmetics

A few formulations are recommended by herbalists for curing general dermatological conditions. These include the use of *Carum copticum* and oral administration of *Piper nigrum* and clarified butter. Thus, a number of medicinal plants and formulations are used for treatment of various dermatological problems. In addition to this, a number of indigenous methods are used for attaining fairness, removing skin dryness and removing dead skin.

5.12.6 Traditional Face Packs and Cosmetics

Face packs and exfoliating scrubs are considered good as these slough away dead cells and impart a fairness glow to the dead skin. These clogs up the top layer of skin and help one look young. Women folk disclosed a number of convention methods employed for the purpose. This includes the use of *batana*, a traditional face pack prepared by grinding kennels of *Prunus armeniaca*, seeds of *Brassica juncea*, *Curcuma longa* rhizome, seeds of *Cicer arietinum* and dried roots of *Valeriana wallichii*. The ingredients are mixed, ground and the paste is rubbed on the face, hands and feet. The rubbing removes the dead skin and imparts a glow to the skin. The use of traditional face pack is very common in marriages and also during festive occasions. The recently available apricot scrubs in the market have drawn idea from conventionally used face packs and scrubs. For instance, the Lotus Apricot scrub available in the market contains paste of apricot kernel, which is also used in the same manner by the people in the region.

Women folk disclosed the use of face pack prepared using seeds of *Lens esculenta,* for which the seeds are soaked overnight in water and ground. The paste is believed to cure oily skin, exfoliates dead skin cells and blackheads, unclogs pores, cleanses facial skin and stimulates skin cells, imparting softness and glow to skin. Women use Fullers' earth or *multani mitti,* which acts as natural skin cleanser, toner and astringent. It is believed to cure oily skin, blemishes and control acne. For removal of unwanted hair, rural women recommend the use of wheat dough, which is gently rubbed on the affected area. A number of indigenous techniques are used for the treatment of dry skin, which includes the application of kernel oil of *Prunus armeniaca*, clarified butter, mixture of mustard oil and wax and milk cream.

5.13 Scalp Conditions

5.13.1 Dandruff or Pityriasis Simplex Capillitii

It is the shedding of dead skin cells from the scalp, caused by frequent exposure to extreme heat and cold. According to local herbalists, the reason of dandruff is disturbance of humoral disturbances which makes the scalp skin dry, resulting in itching of scalp. Conventional treatment involves application of medicated oils along with various herbal preparations, besides adjustments to lifestyle and diet that eliminate the contributing factors. Formulations used for treating dandruff include *Semecarpus anacardium* oil, extract of *Ziziphus jujuba*, juice of *Citrus limon* and gel of *Aloe barbadensis*. For overcoming the balding problem, herbalists recommend the application of fresh gel of *Aloe barbadensis*. Premature greying is treated by using *Sapindus mukorossi* and *Acacia concinna.*

5.13.2 Hair Care Cosmetics

Seeds and leaves of *Sapindus mukorossi* are boiled in water and the extract so prepared is called *choi*. Leaves of *Vitex negundo* and *Adhatoda vasica* are also used for preparing *choi* meant for washing hair. People believe that seeds of *Sapindus mukorossi* have mild insecticidal properties and are traditionally used for eliminating lice from the scalp, besides imparting shine to the hair. Washing hair with buttermilk or curd is recommended by herbalists for imparting shine, removal of dandruff and prevention of hair fall. Indigenous ingredients are used for washing hair, promoting hair growth, prevention of falling hair and premature greying. Traditional hair dyes, fragrant hair rinses are used in the region.

5.13.3 Oral Care

Oral hygiene includes dental care, use of mouth fresheners and lip colouring. But, while looking at modern cosmetic industry, it seems that the whole range of products were conceived and practiced from pre-historic times using the then accessible natural resources. Even today, numerous cosmetics have their origin in the times of yore. The concept of modern day mouth fresheners has evolved from the indigenous systems, which existed among the rural communities. Lips are especially vulnerable to changes in external climatic conditions because the skin is very thin, and hence they are the first to depict the signs of dryness. Lip balm provides an occlusive layer on the lip surface which not only preserves lip moisture but also protect them from external exposure of dry air, cold climatic conditions and winds. A number of indigenous lip guards commonly used include the clotted milk cream, oil of *Prunus armeniaca,* lukewarm clarified butter. Herbalists disclosed that the puckered lips are also cured by applying mustard oil on naval and anus.

Bark of *Juglans regia,* used for cleaning teeth by women folk serve two purposes; it impart reddish shade to the lips and also acts as freshener and cleansing agent. Herbalists recommend the application of *Calotropis gigantean* latex on gums to prevent toothache. Powder of *Syzygium aromaticum* buds and *Piper nigrum* seeds, dried flowers of *Anacyclus Pyrethrum* with water are recommended for the same problem. Stem of *Zanthoxylum armatum* is used as tooth cleaner and mouth freshener.

5.13.4 Cosmetics for Hands and Feet

For softening hands and feet, women folk in tribal areas, apply oil of *Prunus armeniaca*. Besides this, they make use of clotted milk-cream for the same purpose. A unique method of treating cracked heels, include the filling the same with the resin of *Cedrus deodara,* followed by pressing it with a pair of hot tongs. The hot metallic touch not only melts and fills the resin in cracks but also provide relief to aching heels.

5.14 Snake and Insect Bite

Treatment of snakebites had assumed importance since times immemorial. Services of traditional healers have been sought by people in remote localities where modern anti-venom treatment has not reached. But nowadays, a holistic approach is adopted, where modern antivenin based treatment and practices of traditional healers are combined. There are a few healers who specially deal in removal of poison from the body. This may include the poison of plant or animal origin but the emphasis is on snake/scorpion poison. The treatment involves the use of few concoctions along with magico-religious therapy. The method of treatment is kept secret and is passed on from one generation to other, for instance, in *Kinnaur*; a woman who treats snake bite poisoning has inherited the art of healing from her father and uses her spit for the treatment. The spit is applied on the affected area. During the visit to the village where she lives, people narrated that a number of patients from within state and outside visit her for the treatment.

A variety of formulations including pastes and extracts are used for treating insect and snake bites. Extract of *Cannabis sativa* mixed with kerosene oil is suggested for local application on the affected area. Paste of *Nux vomica* or extract of *Ficus religosa* leaves and *Achyranthes aspera* or paste of Serpentine stone is used by the folk healers. Victim of snake bite is made to consume kerosene oil to reduce the effect of poison in the body.

Magical healing is also done in case of insect or snake bite. In this, not only the poison is removed but also the shock and after effects of bite is cured. At times, combinations of herbal drugs are also given to the patient along with '*jhadha*' which is usually done with chanting of '*mantras*'.

Achyranthes aspera is highly esteemed by traditional healers and used in the treatment of scorpion bite, snake bite and skin diseases, etc. (Jain 1991).Traditional healers claim that addition of *A. aspera* enhances the efficacy of any drug of plant origin. Scientists have reported properties of *Nux vomica* like that of alkaloid strychnine and its use as an antidote in various types of poisoning. *Nux vomica* is used by traditional healers in curing poisoning caused by insect or snake bites.

5.15 Generalized Health Problems

Treatments for general health problems such as metabolic disorders (diabetes), fever, headache and allergies is also done by the traditional healers. They classify fever into several varieties depending upon the vitiation of the three *doshas* namely, *vata*, *pitta*, and *kapha*; the change of climate or seasons; the vitiation of the vital fluid, blood and other supplementary reasons. For treating fever of any kind, the use of decoctions is recommended. The main herbal constituents of these decoctions are *Tracheyspermum ammi*, *Emblica officinalis*, *Terminalia bellirica*, *Terminalia chebula* and *Ocimum sanctum*. For treating malaria fever, decoction of *Ocimum sanctum*, *Piper nigrum* and sugar in water is suggested by healers, whereas in tribal areas, *Inula racemosus* and *Sascussurea costus* are used for curing fever. Local application of paste of *Eucalyptus* is recommended for getting relief from headache. Role of *Tracheyspermum ammi, Terminalia chebula, Ocimum sanctum* and *Piper nigrum* in treatment of fever has also been described in *Ayurveda* and other traditional medicines.

5.16 Ear Nose and Throat Problems

A common auditory affliction is an ache in the ear, which may be due to acute inflammation in the middle ear or due to chronic inflammation, boils, eczema, wax, or decay in a tooth. These problems are treated by using certain formulations including extracts, oils or pastes which are either administered orally or applied locally on the affected areas. For curing ear-ache, the healers suggest the extract of leaves of *Delphinium denudatum*, extract of *Channa orientalis* stem, extract of *Agave americana*, extract of *Calendula officinalis* flower, etc. Dropping of lukewarm oil boiled with *Zingiber officinale* is also recommended in certain areas of the state. In *Kinnaur*, for treating, ear aches, oil of *Prunus armeniaca* kennel is dropped in the ears and plugged with cotton. Mumps, a disease which affects the parotid salivary glands and results in the swelling of glands, high fever and headache, are treated with a number of applications prepared using *Sapindussp., Piper nigrum*, *Zingiber officinale*, *Syzygium aromaticum* and *Capsicumannuum*. For treating mumps, healers suggest:

> …Kernel of *Sapindes mukerossi* and seeds of *Piper nigrum* are ground in water and the paste is applied on the affected area. Local application of lukewarm paste of *Aloe barbadensis, Zingiber officinale* powder, *Syzgium aromaticum, Cinamomum zeylaricum,* extract of *Trachyspermum ammi,* and *Linum usitatissimum* prepared in cow urine is also effective for the same problem.

Tonsillitis, an inflammation of lymphoid tissues behind the tongue, on either side of the pharynx is treated by orally administering powder of seeds of *Nelumbo nucifera*, *Acacia catechu*, extract of *Bambusa sp.*, *Elettaria cardamonum* and *borax* powder. Healers suggest its administration with lukewarm water before sunrise in the morning and before sunset in the evening. Minor gums and teeth problems are handled by application of latex of *Calotropis gigantean*, powder of *Piper nigrum*, *Red Ocher*, Copper sulphate and ammonium chloride on the affected area.

5.17 Eye Care

The organs of sight, eyes, are the most delicate part of the body. Conjunctivitis, an inflammation of the conjunctiva or mucous membrane connecting the inner eyelid and eyeball, is a common eye infection which results in redness of the eye. It is common among people whose eyes are exposed to dust, smoke, cold and winds.

For treating conjunctivitis or redness in eyes, herbalists recommend application of paste of *Pterocarpus santalinus*and *Terminalia chebula* on eyes, besides putting drops of honey, and extract of rose flower. A special type of paste is suggested for reducing redness of the eyes. For this, *rasont* (prepared from the roots of *Berberis aristata*) is mixed in breast milk of women undergone parturition and the paste is applied on the eyes. Another traditional ointment for same problem is prepared by rubbing dried umbilical cord and copper coin in mother's milk. The ointment is applied on affected eyes. For curing conjunctivitis, elderly women suggest, application of fresh milk cream on eyes on which the slices of cucumber are placed and the patient is allowed to lie down for an hour. Ancient scriptures mention that the roots of *Barberis aristata* possess antibacterial and anti-inflammatory properties and hence used in the treatment of painful eye affectations.

5.18 Urinary Problems

According to herbalists, improper functioning of different *doshas* of body results in formation of kidney stones and causes pain and inflammation in the kidney. A number of formulations are used for urinary problems. These medicinal preparations contain *Hordeum vulgare*, ammonium nitrate, *Dolichos biflorus* seeds, ammonium chloride, leaves of *Bergenia ligulata*, *Ziziphus sp.* fruit, *Coleus amboinicus* and *Fumaria parviflora* in different combinations. The preparations are mainly in the form of decoctions, tablets or extracts. Herbalist suggests that application of castor oil on abdominal region removes kidney stone. Oral administration of decoction prepared by using bark of *Bauhinia variegata* tree in water is beneficial for getting rid of kidney stones. Extract of *Cucumis melo* if taken empty stomach, relieves the pain of renal calculi. Researchers have reported that among various medicines, *Bergenia ligulata* has a high reputation in indigenous systems of medicine for dissolving stones in the kidneys.

5.19 Managing Diabetes

Diabetes is one of the major public health problems presently affecting 284.6 million people globally and according to recent International Diabetes Federation (IDF) estimations it is likely to influence 438.4 million people by 2030 becoming one of the world's main disabler and killer (IDF 2009). According to the World Health Organisation estimates, India had 32 million diabetic subjects in the year 2000 and this number would increase to 80 million by the year 2030 (Wild et al. 2004). Type 1 diabetes is described by poor insulin production and needs daily administration of insulin, while Type 2 diabetes results from the body's ineffective use of insulin. The cause of type 1 diabetes is not known and it is not preventable with current knowledge, whereas Type 2 diabetes comprises 90 % of

Table 5.3 Plants used for the treatment of diabetes

Scientific name	Vernacular name	Part used
Swertia chirayata	Chirayata	Leaves
Momoydica sp.	Kerale	Seeds
Cassia angustifolia	Sanaya	Leaves
Vinca rosea	Sadabahar	Leaves
Azadirachsta indica	Neem	Leaves
Syzygium cuminii	Jamum	Seeds
Cinnamomum tamala	Tejpatar	Leaves
Trigonelia sp.	Kasuri methi	Leaves
Ocimum sanctum	Tulsi	Leaves
Withania somnifera	Ashvangadha	Leaves
Trigonella foenum	Methi	Leaves
Curcuma longa	Haldi	Rhizome
Papaver somniferum	Afimdana	Seeds
Prunus dulcis	Badam	Seeds
Ajuja biacteosa	Neelkanthi	Leaves
Terminalia chebula	Harad	Fruit
Terminalia bellirica	Bhera	Fruit
Emblica officinalis	Amla	Fruit
Pandanus odoratissimus	Kewda	Flower
Gymnema sylvestre	Gudmaar	Leaves
Mangnifera indica	Amb	Kernel

people with diabetes around the world, and is mainly the consequence of excess body weight and immobility (Cerqueira 2010). Although it is the type 2 diabetes which is more widespread and the main driver of diabetes epidemic in India, it is noted that occurrence of type 1 diabetes in India is also on the rise (Ramachandran et al. 1995). Due to convenience and cultural acceptance, more than 80 % of the population in some Asian and African countries relies on traditional medicines and Traditional Health Practitioners (THPs) for primary health care (WHO 2002a, b). However, the information on local plants used conventionally in Himachal Himalayas for the management of diabetes mellitus is inadequate. A few plants recommended for treating diabetes mellitus are (Table 5.3).

These plants are used individually or in combination, for instance, the leaves of *Vinca rosea* and *Gymnema sylvestre* are consumed individually, while leaves of *Swertia chirayata,* kernel of *Syzygium cuminii, Prunus dulcis fruit* and *Papaver somniferum* seeds are used in combination.

5.20 Traditional Orthopedic Practitioners

Traditional orthopaedic practices are one of the key branches of traditional medicine especially in rural and inaccessible areas, which have relived people from the orthopaedic conditions. These include wide range of practices such as managing of fracture, dislocation, primary care of patients experiencing chronic musculoskeletal and neurological conditions.

The traditional orthopaedic practitioners have an understanding of vital body points, including bones and joints, specialized massaging techniques and herbal medicinal preparations for speedy healing of injury. There are healers who specialize in bone-setting, setting fractures, handling dislocations and sprains. The traditional bone-setters are dependent on the touch of their hands. They, with the help of their fingers investigate and recognize the affected area and are able to place and pull the concerned limbs and joints, thereby relocating the bones. The bonesetters use small pieces of earthen ware, or even mud to give support to affected areas which include use of available wood as casts.They also make use of use traditional bandages or slings made from locally available wood and woollen cloth. Most of them use herbal ointments and medicated oils which they smear on wounds to hasten the process of healing. Mostly the art of bone setting and managing of sprains and dislocation is inherited as a family tradition and in some cases the skills are imparted by teachers through casual apprenticeship.

The bone setter and practitioners dealing with neuro-muscular disorders are easily accessible, highly skilled in management of simple fractures, are cost effective and make use of medicated oils and pastes which has faster healing effect and strengthens the musculature at fracture location. Revitalising the accessible science of bone-setting would be a gainful alternative for the costly "state of the art" contemporary techniques, especially in the mountainous areas. Numerous herbs are used for preparation of splints, poultices, medicated oils, etc. The massage men of *Shikari Devi* in district Mandi for treating slip-disc and bone-setter of Hamirpur are well known for their specialized art of healing throughout the state. The herbalists of Naarag, Sayree and Dhundan in district Solan are well-recognized for handling paralytic patients.

Formulations have been documented for the treatment of various musculo-skeletal disorders. These formulations are available for back ache/joint pains, paralysis, disc problem, general body aches, bone setting, etc. This includes various types of decoctions and powders for oral administration and application of pastes/oils on affected areas (Table 5.4).

The formulations meant for handling neuro-muscular disorders contain a number of ingredients; some of them are *Zingiber officinale*, *Cynodondactylon*, *Tribulus terrestris*, *Curcuma longa*, *Cinnamomum comphora* and *Sesamum indicum* oil. In addition to medicines of plant origin, some constituents of animal origin are also included in the treatment of musculoskeletal disorders e.g. fish oil dissolved in milk is suggested for oral administration; powder of *Nemorhaedus goral* horn's is recommended for oral administration. Application of animal fat is suggested for back ache, joint pain and paralysis. Massage of *Sesamum indicum* oil is advised for treatment of paralysis. Along with herbal medicines, some traditional procedures are also employed for treating musculoskeletal disorders. Bloodletting is done for treating general body aches, swelling and inflammation (Figs. 5.1 and 5.2). For this, a hole is made on the tip of a buffalo horn and the horn

Table 5.4 Formulation used for neuro-muscular disorders

Problem	Formulations recommended by bonesetter/folk orthopaedic practitioners
Back ache/joint pain	Local application of *Sesamum indicum* oil on affected area
	Decoction of *Zingiber officinale, Trigonella foenum, Curcuma longa* and *Tribulus terrestris* for oral administration
	Application of paste of *Curcuma longa, Emblica officinalis, Cynodondactylon* and *Capsicum annuum* on the affected area
	Seeds of *Datura metel, Pipernigrum, Piper longum, Zingiber officinale,* and *Trachyspermum ammi* are grinded and mixed with extract of *Zingiber officinale*; followed by preparation of its tablets. Tablets are orally administered with warm water
	Seeds of *Cuminum cyminum* are dried, parched and grinded. The powder is recommended with milk
	Seeds of Lepidium sativum are dried roasted and recommended with milk
	Seeds of Eruca vesicaria are roasted and grinded, followed by addition of salt to this powder. Powder is given with water
	Fish oil dissolved in milk is suggested for oral administration
	Horns of *Nemorhaedus goral* are grinded and powder is orally administered with hot milk
	Vespa sp. is made to bite the aching joints so as to induce poison in the body. The sting is believed to provide relief to the aches
	Animal fat of *Ursus sp.* is heated and melted fat is used for massaging the affected areas.
	Melted animal fat of *Capra hircus* is applied on affected area
	Saussurea costus is grinded, mixed in kennel oil of *Prunus armeniaca* and recommended for local application on affected area
	Application of animal fat of *Cannis sp.* boiled/heated on affected area.
	Local application of kennel oil of *Prunus armeniaca* on affected area.
	Oral administration of powder of *Berberis aristata* roots with water
Paralysis	Massage with *Sesamum indicum* oil
	Leaves of *Vitex negundo, Datura metal, Acorus calamus, Zingiber officinale, Mentha piperita*, and C*innamomum camphora* are added to *Sesamum indicum* oil. The oil so prepared is applied on the affected area after hot water fomentation
	Leaves of *Vitex negundo, Mentha piperita, Eucalyptus globulus* and *Cuscuta reflexa* together with cow urine, rock salt are boiled in water. The medicated water so prepared is used for fomentation
Disc problem	*Stephania glabra*, leaves of *Vitex negundo Gentiana kurroo, Cuscuta reflexa, Adhatoda vasica, Azadirachta indica* and *Alum* are boiled in cow urine and water till the mixture is reduced to half. Oil of *Sesamum indicum* is added to this along with ground *Syzgium aromaticum*, Myristica fragrans and C*innamomum camphora.* The oil so prepared is applied on affected area
Bone setting	Fresh *Curcuma longa* and rock salt are grinded and the paste is applied on the affected area
Sciatic pain	Local application of fish oil on affected area

is touched with the affected area and suction is done. Then an incision is given on the affected area and blood is allowed to come out. It is believed that bloodletting relieves body pain and reduces swelling.

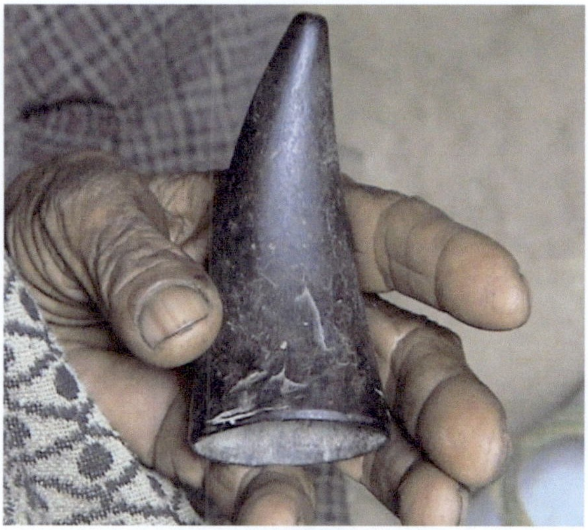

Fig. 5.1 Buffalo horn used for blood letting

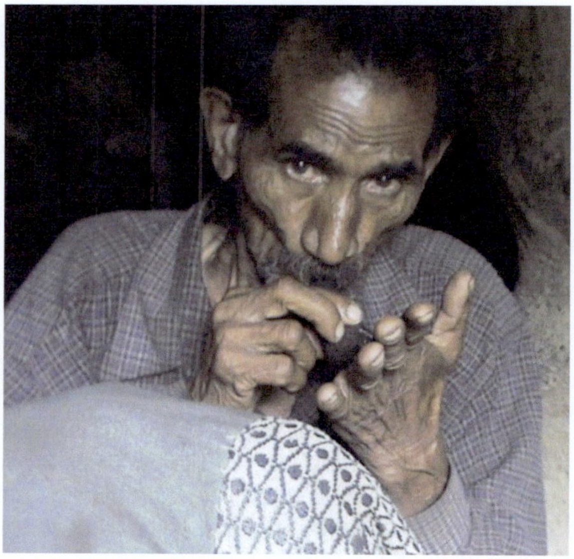

Fig. 5.2 Blood letting expert depicting the procedure

In yet another such procedure followed for relieving joint pains, an incision is made on the affected area and after bloodletting, latex of *Calotropis gigantean* is applied on the wound. The wound is covered for some days and formation of pus is allowed. Thereafter, the pus is removed and it is believed that removing the pus relieves the pain. For treating sciatic pain, patient's leg is tied with rope and then an incision is given between thumb and fist finger of foot to allow bloodletting which relieves the pain.

Use of *Sesamum indicum* oil for joint pains finds mention in *Ayurveda*, where its role is described in treating gout and inflammations (Kulkarni 2000). *Cinnamomum camphor* has a long history of herbal use but it is mainly used as essential oil. Bown (1995) reported its similar use in creams for treating joint and muscle pains. *Sasussurea costus* is also used in *Ayurvedic* medicine where it is mainly valued for its nutritive, stimulant and antiseptic properties. The root is anodyne, antibacterial, antispasmodic, stimulant, stomachic, tonic and vermifuge. It is used internally in the treatment of body pains (Kulkarni 2000). Though this can prove to be a profitable profession, most bonesetters have maintained a low profile and charge no or very less fee. Each patient donates what he can afford as an offering. These institutions are rendering valuable service to the people living in tough areas of Himalayan region; many of them are tribals, farmers and nomads who cannot afford costly treatment in a modern hospital.

5.21 Managing Gastrointestinal Disorders

A number of disorders are associated with the functioning of digestive system. These include diarrhoea, or frequent evacuation of bowels; gastritis or inflammation of the stomach which eventually gives rise to many life-threatening complications, if not treated in time. The most common disorder is, perhaps, constipation. If constipation continues for some time, it may lead to a feeling of heaviness of abdomen and later headaches, lethargy and loss of appetite and even piles. According to herbalists, the main causes of piles are chronic constipation, obesity, mental tension and hereditary factors. Herbalists reported piles as a cause of low digestive fire.

In almost all the formulations meant for treatment of digestive disorders, *Mentha longifolia* is used along with *Cuminum cyminum*, *Nelimbo nucifera*, *Mesua ferrea, Allium cepa*, *Syzygium aromaticum* and *Zingiber officinale*. Roots of *Podophyllum hexandrum* are used for controlling nausea. *Ayurveda* mentions various properties of *Cuminum cyminum*. It is hot, sweet, cooling, antihelmentic, carminative and anti-dysenteric. It acts as an astringent to bowels and helps in controlling belching. It has been demonstrated scientifically that ingestion of *Zingiber officinale* is one of the best remedies to combat nausea and vomiting.

Formulations for handling gastric problems contain *Terminalia chebula, Terminalia bellirica* and *Emblica officinalis* as the basic constituents in addition to *Cassia angustifolia*, *Carum copticum* and black salt. In tribal areas, the main constituent of almost all the formulation recommended for treating gastric, contains *Bunium persicum* along with *Cuminum cyminum* and *Zingiber officinale*. For treating preliminary stage of gastric ulcers, herbalists recommend the oral administration of latex of *Euphorbia royleana* plant. In *Ayurveda*, *Terminalia chebula, Terminalia bellirica*, *Emblica officinalis* are the main constituents of *trifala* which is known to enhance the thirteen digestive fires. The preparations used for treating constipation usually contain *Cassia angustifolia* as the main constituent along with *Terminalia sp.* and *Rosa sp.,* extracts of *Tinospora cordifolia* and pulp of *Cassia fistula.* In tribal areas of Himachal, decoction of *Picrorhiza kurooa* and *Aconitum hetrophyllum* is given for treating constipation.

The formulations used for treating jaundice and liver problems contain *Nelumbo nucifera*, *Piper longum* and *Ficus religiosa*. Extract of *Ficus religiosa* leaf, mixed with honey is recommended for jaundice and liver problems. In tribal areas, powder of *Bunium persicum* is used in treatment of jaundice. Herbalists also recommend a variety of treatments for worm infestation. Most of the medicinal preparations for the purpose are recommended with curd or butter milk and preferably empty stomach. Use of *Brassica juncea*, *Ficus carica*, *Hyoscymus niger*, *Adium graveolems* and *Myrica nagi* in various combinations is recommended. In tribal areas, *Bunium persicum*is advised empty stomach with lukewarm water for the removal of worms.

A number of preparations are suggested for treating dysentery. These are mainly in the form of decoctions and powders. Some of the common plants used by the folk herbalists for the purpose are *Anethum graveolens*, *Terminalia chebula*, *Bunium persicum*, *Aegle marmelos*, *Corriandrum sativum*, *Plantago ovata* and *Papaver somriferum*. For treatment of blood stools, powder of *Foeniculum valgare*, *Cuminum cyminum*, *Plantago ovata* and *Papaver somniferum* is recommended. Decoction of dried *Aconitum heterophyllum* is suggested for the same problem. The formulations used for curing stomach-ache include *Trachyspermum sp.* and *Terminalia sp.* Healers revealed:

> ...We recommend tying of *Ricinus communis* leaves on stomach after heating, for getting relief from stomach-ache. Local application of *Ferula asafoetida* melted in ghee on affected area is also beneficial...

In Kinnaur, decoction *Aconitum heterophyllum* roots and powder of *Picrorrhiza kurrooa* is recommended by herbalists for stomach-ache. Scientific studies reported *Ferula asafetida* as effective medicinal herb used in the *Ayurvedic* tradition that acts mainly on the digestive system and helps in cleansing and strengthening of gastro-intestinal tract. *Picrorhiza kurrooa* is a well-known plant employed to treat a number of ailments in traditional medicinal systems of Bhutan, China, India and Nepal (Anon 1993; Tsarong 1986). The plant is regarded as being one of the major components of *Arogyavardhini*, a potent *Ayurvedic* formulation used to treat liver ailments (Kapahi et al. 1993). Studies have shown that *Picrorhiza kurrooa* has curative effect for fever, malnutrition due to digestive disturbance, jaundice, diarrhoea and dysentery (Zhang and Zhang 1994).

Piles according to traditional healers are caused due to low digestive fire which results in accumulation of digestive impurities or toxins that aggravates the *doshas* in rectal canal, leading to internal or external piles. Various preparations used for treating piles include the oral administration or local application of medicinal preparations. Most of the preparations contain *Piper nigrum* along with *Curcuma longa*, *Sphaerantus indices* and *Calendula officinalis*. A healer revealed the local application of paste of grinded moulting of snake skin in mustard oil for effectively treating the problem

For treating general disorders of stomach, oral administration of tablets prepared by making use of leaves of *Wattakaka volubilis* and molasses is recommended by traditional healers. Local application of sheep milk is recommended for the treatment of mouth ulcers in many areas of Himachal. Thus, a number of diseases affecting the digestive system are cured by healers using the locally available curative herbs.

5.22 Handling Respiratory Disorders

Cough, bronchitis, asthma, and pneumonia are some of the common respiratory disorders. Bronchitis is characterized by inflammation of the bronchial tubes which carry air to the lungs. According to folk herbalists, cold and cough is caused by aggravation of *kaphadosha*. It may sometimes be due to weak digestion. When the food is not fully digested it changes into mucus, which gets mixed with various circulations and reaches the respiratory system causing cold or cough. Important constituents in almost all decoctions and powders used for treating cold are *Zingiber officinale*, *Viala serpens*, *Cinamomum zeylenium*, *Elettaria cardamonum*, *Glyeentrize glabra* and *Foeniculum vulgare*. In the formulations used for the treatment of cough, *Viala serpens*, *Pistacia integerrima*, *Piper nigrum* and *Piper longum* are the main constituents. These constituents are known for their curative value especially in curing cough and cold. In all formulations meant for asthma, *Achyranthes aspera*, *Vitis sp.*, *Commiphora guggul*, *Pistacia integerrima* and *Ficus religosa* are the main constituents.

In tribal areas, powder of *Bunium persicum* is given with warm water for treating cough and cold. Besides this, local wine proves to be beneficial for overcoming the respiratory problems. The use of *Glyeentrize glabra* in treatment of Addison's disease, asthma, bronchitis and cough has been reported by number of researchers. *Elettaria cardamonum* is described as a potent bronchodilator in *Ayurveda* (Sharma and Dash 2002).

5.23 World of Traditional Birth Attendants

For most women, the period between puberty and menopause offer multiple opportunities for personal realization and development. Yet, this can also be a time of health risks particularly associated with sex and reproduction that may result in a considerable burden of mortality and disability (WHO 2009). Complications of pregnancy and childbirth are major causes of death and disability among women of reproductive age in developing countries. Every day at least 1,600 women die from the complications of pregnancy and childbirth (Tinker et al. 2000).

According to an estimate of World Health Organization (WHO), approximately 80 % of the people in developing countries depend on traditional medicines for primary health care needs and majority of these involves the use of plants due to accessibility and cultural acceptance (WHO 2005). The conventional procedures and medicine advised by the venerable birth attendants is said to have a long and respectable history—much longer than contemporary western medicine. Its roots are embedded in antiquity (Bright 2000). In older times, and even today, the conventional knowledge and practices remained the basis for the wellbeing and livelihoods of indigenous women, maintaining their health and also in reinstating their socio-cultural milieu. The Himalayan region is rich in resource wealth as well as indigenous wisdom. How the traditional wisdom evolved is not known to anybody, but it is believed that gossips and fallacies formed the basis of transmission of this knowledge. But, it remained confined to practitioners and few beneficiaries, and later on became more concealed and less accessible to general public (Abbink 1995). In Himachal Himalayas, several medicinal plants are traditionally used to manage gynaecological problems. However, information on local medicinal plants used traditionally for the said purpose is scare. With the passage of time the conventional knowledge on various aspects of women's health is on a decline and younger generation is showing least concern in learning this art of healing.

Traditional birth attendants are often familiarized with the socio-cultural backdrop of mother, which enables them to offer psychological support to mother. However, in earlier times, the birthing process in tribal areas of *Kinnaur* was facilitated by male birth attendants locally called *Amchi*, or the traditional medicine men, who were capable in handling delivery. They practiced the profession in the unapproachable areas, where medical aid could not be provided. Women in tribal district of Kinnaur narrated, that earlier, the women in labor use to carry out the delivery by herself, for which she was kept isolated in a cowshed.

The birth attendants in Himachal Himalayas are of two types—the herbalist engaged in midwifery and others limiting to midwifery only. They hold a position of power and authority among Himalayan communities. They adhere to specific dietary rules and consequently act as predominant spreaders of ideas related to the type and effect of food. Their wisdom help them in relieving the uneasiness and distress of mothers during pregnancy, speeding up of birthing process, prevention of bleeding as well as in inducing abortion if necessary, treatment of dysmenorrhoea and related illnesses. They provide prenatal and post-natal care, which is usually in the form of guidance regarding food consumption. They restrict certain eatables and activities. The guidance regarding the reproductive health is usually shaped and strengthened by local beliefs and practices, most of which are governed by spiritual or mystic traditions, for instance, the women during her menstrual cycle is not allowed to enter in kitchen or sacred place for at least 5 days. This is considered unclean period during which she is allowed to take rest. A woman is generally restricted from attending religious rituals and social interactions during menstrual cycle or birthing. These beliefs and practices are still prevalent among the Himalayan communities. Another customary practice prevalent in the state is that during the postpartum period mother and baby are kept in isolation for at least 16 days. Mother can enter the kitchen and sacred place only after the ritual bath. Burying of umbilical cord and placenta at the place of delivery is culturally considered a significant ritual.

5.23.1 Knowledge of Handling Gynaecological Problems and Birthing

The interviewees had good knowledge of clinical symptoms related to gynecological problems particularly menstrual disorders, infertility, repeated abortions, leucorrhea, etc. and management of labor. In addition to advising herbal remedies for getting relief from aches, illness or distress, the midwifes advise unique massages. They have evolved their own conventional methods to foretell the date of delivery. During the parturition these attendants assist mothers in speeding up the expulsion of baby, removal of placenta and management of bleeding. These interventions include application of heat or substances to mother's abdomen or birth canal, maintenance of special postures, use of outer pressure on the abdomen, dilatation of vagina, oral administration of special herbal teas or decoctions to expedite labor or to stop bleeding. After the birth, the midwife cuts and ties the umbilical cord. They often provide help in cooking special food for mothers and washing their clothes. They also assist in mother's ritual bath and looking after of newborn. There is no restriction or interference with the practices and procedures adopted by birth attendants. An assortment of decoctions, herbal extracts, powders, etc., are recommended for oral intake and local application. Most of them, having the knowledge of identifying plant and its usage are also expert in preparing formulations. They precisely know about the collecting and processing herbs, requirement of herbs for preparing formulations, time required as well as the method of application. The decoctions are mainly prepared by boiling the herbs in water or milk. While many herbs are dried, grinded and stored in powdered form, while a few are used in fresh form Herbalists, traditional midwife and elderly women recommend numerous formulations for treating gynecological disorders and birthing. A variety of locally available plants, for instance, *Quercus infectoria, Bombax cebia, Cannabis sativa,* etc. are the ingredients of these formulations. Infertility is the unusual state of a woman where she is unable to carry a pregnancy to full term because of certain biological cause (Tables 5.5 and 5.6).

In India, oil of *Acoruscalamus* is given to haemorrhaging women after an abortion (Dastur 1951). Mixed with saffron and mare's milk, it is administered to hasten delivery during childbirth (Dastur 1951). Infusion of bark of *Anogeissus latifolia* is given for easy delivery (Kamble et al. 2010). It is also used to cure the damaged tissue during delivery (Meena and Rao 2010). *Asparagus racemosus* is used for treating excess bleeding during menstrual discharge and burning sensation in urine (Shukla et al. 2008). It promotes fertility, reduce menstrual cramping, and increase milk production in nursing mothers (Negi et al. 2010). Leaves of *Bombax ceiba* are used for leucorrhoea, anaemia, infertility. Flowers are used for anaemia, leucorrhoea, gonorrhoea and menstrual disorders (Verma et al. 2011). Seeds of *Bryonopsis laciniosa* are used to cure sterility/ impotency and used as a tonic in women (Arjariya and Chaurasia 2009; Ehsan et al 2009). *Glycyrrhiza glabra* is a tonic, anti-inflammatory, Anti-biotic, aphrodisiac, prescribed for promoting lactation (Nalini and Thomas 2009) and is used in the treatment of sex-hormone imbalances and

Table 5.5 Plant species reported by traditional midwives and herbalists for managing infertility

Botanical name	Vernacular name
Quercus infectoria	Majuphal
Sida cordifolia	Dhreed
Bombax cebia	Mochras
Anogeissus latifolia	Dhav
Coriandrum sativum	Dhaniya
Mesua ferrea	Nagkesar
Acoruscalamus	Vach
Terminalia chebula	Bari harad
Withania somnifera	Ashwagndha
Myrsine africana	Vaibiding
Holarrhena antidysenterica	Kurakadi
Cannabis sativa	Bhang
Anethum graveolens	Kadvi saunf
Cynodon dactylon	Dhruv
Acacia catechu	Supari
Glycerrhiza glabra	Mulethi
Mesua ferrea	Nagkesar
Ipomoea digitata	Vidarikand
Nelumbonucifera	Tal makahanna
Chlorophytum borivilianum	Safedmusli
Asparagus racemosus	Satavari
Mucuna pruriens	Kauch
Piper nigrum	Kali Mirch

Table 5.6 Formulations reported by traditional midwives for managing gynaecological problems

Childbirth Fever (*Prasuti Jwara*)	Decoction of *Nardostachys grandiflora, Boswellia serrata, Santalum album,* powder and *Sentella asiatica* is recommended for oral administration
General Gynaecological problems	Oral administration ofdecoction of *Oryza sativa*, *Bambusa sp*, *Butea Monosperma*, *Asparagus racemosus*, *Cynodon dactylon*, and *Acacia catechu*
	Dried roots and leaves of *Sida cordifolia* are grinded and kept in an earthen vessel along with some water. The mixture is stirred with the help of *Justicia adhatondo* stem. The liquid is filtered and given to the patient
Blood purification of a pregnant woman	7 to 8 Seeds of *Piper nigrum* are grinded mixed with clarified butter and sugar and recommended for oral administration
Repeated abortions	Seeds of *Bryonopsis* laciniosa are recommended for oral administration
Leucorrhoea	Ash of dry epicarp of *Cocos nucifera is* suggested for oral administration

menopausal symptoms in women (Gupta et al. 2008). For curing menstrual problem, seed powder of *Mesua ferrea* is recommended with pepper and milk (Shivanna and Rajkumar 2010). *Sida cordifolia* is tonic, astringent, emollient, aphrodisiac treats Gonorrhea, frequent micturition and Leucorrhoea. Seeds are particularly considered as aphrodisiac (Jain et al. 2011). Root of *Withania somnifera* are used for the treatment of infertility, impotence, repeated miscarriage, paralysis, memory loss, multiple sclerosis (Bhagwan 1991). These studies are thus concurrent with the usage pattern adopted by the traditional healers of North-western Himalayas.

5.24 *Amchis*: Traditional Healers of Kinnaur

Tribal communities of *Kinnaur* have developed their own healthcare system based on the availability of natural resources and the knowledge inherited from ancestors. This system of healing is known as the *Amchi* system of healing. The word *amchi,* derived from *bhoti* language means 'superior to all'. The *amchis* do not merely follow ancient manuscripts, but also have practical knowledge on preparing medicines. The traditional knowledge, practices and beliefs of *amchis* remained undocumented, and passed on from one generation to the next by word of mouth (Fig. 5.3). *Amchis* enjoy great respect and high social status among the communities living in *Kinnaur*. But, they are apprehensive of phasing out of the tradition with the penetration of modern facilities in remote corners of the state. In order to pass on their valuable knowledge and practices, they are keen to teach the eager and deserving learners. In Kinnaur, *Amchi* knowledge is imparted through some social institutions. In the monastery of Sangla, it is imparted to students by monks. Here, group learning helps them in sharing of knowledge on medicinal plants and also help in spreading the knowledge across different villages in the district. While interviewing traditional healers from *Kinnaur* it was found that there is a lot of vagueness in the nomenclature of plants used. In practice, these practitioners use different names for the same plant and sometimes one name for different plant species. In old manuscripts, plant names and its ethno-medical significance is well defined. This system of medicine involves the use of proper diagnostic skills based on the vision, and consideration of practitioner. The system takes into account the key principles of Buddhism i.e. humanity, karma and moral values. *Amchi* principles are catalogued in an organized and reasonable framework based on an understanding of the body and its relationship with the environment.

The *Amchi* system involves the use of numerous treatment methods of curing disease. The treatment can be done by suggesting balance diet, medication and physical healing. Of the various techniques used for treatment, puncturing of body part or veins is most important. This method is used for curing headache, paralysis, inflammation of joints, arthritis, etc. Depending upon the type and seriousness of disease, flower heads of some plants, animal horns, needles of iron, gold, or silver are used of puncturing. These needles are heated and touched with affected area. Veins are punctured in such a manner to allow the outflow of blood. The needles or

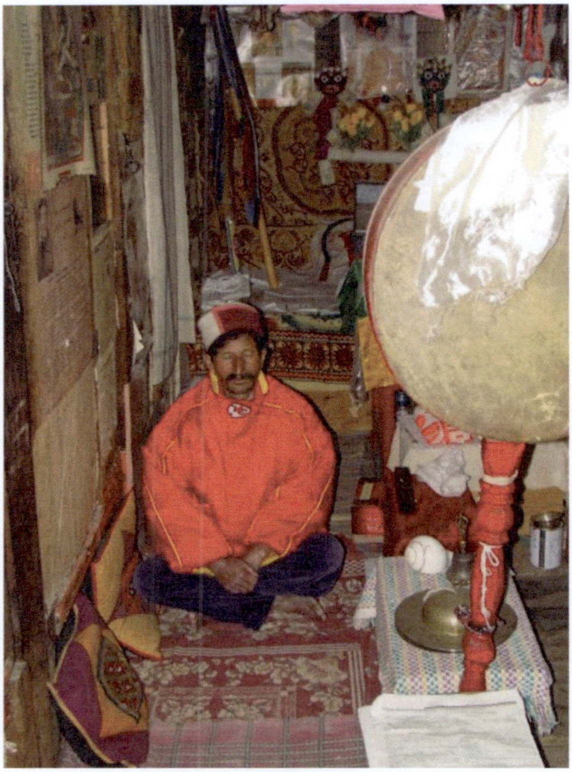

Fig. 5.3 Amchi traditional medicine man

wires are used to treat the brain related disorders such as epilepsy. Heated needles are touched at specific points time and again. Initially the patient feels some pain but with the passage of time, this pain fades out. Placing of needle on body parts requires special skill which one learns with experience. Special points are marked for touching the needle.

Though the material of vegetal origin is the chief component of medicine, products of animal origin, and minerals and salts are also used for preparing medicines. Minerals include gold, silver, copper, iron, *shilajeet*, rock salt, etc. Formulations are prepared by using number of ingredients. The medicinal formulations are in form of tablets, concoctions, decoctions or powder. Animal body parts are used for treating various ailments. Horns, flesh, blood, urine, hair, faecal matter, bones, skin, etc. are used. The animals whose body parts/excretions are used for preparing medicines are antelopes, rhinoceros, wild and domestic sheep, pig, dog, fox, sparrow, peacock, deer, yak, ass, snake, horse, cow, pigeon, beer, musk deer, snow leopard, etc.

Wild plants are used for preparing medicines, and at times, these plants are toxic and poisonous. Different parts of plants such as roots, stem, bark, leaves, flowers, fruits and tubers are used for the purpose.

Amchi system of medicine is gradually declining in Kinnaur, because new generations are not showing their interest in this art of healing. Older generations had good knowledge of plants and their identification, but the coming generations don't feel like visiting the field to be trained in identification of plants. However, it is commendable on part of government, some NGOs and various *Amchis* who are making sincere efforts to keep the tradition alive. With the establishment of *Amchis* Training Centres in Dharmshala, Darjeeling, Ladakh and Manali, many people are showing interest in this system and undertaking proper training courses conducted at these centres. A few Associations and *Amchi* Institutes are trying to popularize this system of medicine and as a result the system is gaining momentum in the modern world. A Tibetan Medical School and Central Institute (TMAI) has been established at Dharmshala to continue and disseminate the traditional knowledge. Some other non-governmental organizations are focusing on conservation and promotion of *Amchi* system of medicine and popularizing this age-old tradition at global level. But, these systems require appreciation, revival, reverence and thoughtful consideration. The utmost challenge is integration of conventional knowledge with contemporary.

The process of healing is deeply embedded in the culture of North-Western Himalayas. The conceptual cost of sickness, diagnosis, treatment and other interaction are important in understanding and managing sickness. Sickness is a fundamental physical attack on person and society and is a matter of deepest human concern. It implies that the experience of healing is highly marked. When patient experiences some pain and goes to healer for a diagnosis, the healer after diagnosis suggests the treatment. The strategy a person chooses for the treatment of his or her illness or that of a relative depends on personal experiences and preferences. The community's response to health problems reveals a multiple and simultaneous usage of home remedies and multiple therapy. The practitioners whose services are sought are Gods and Goddesses, local deities, folk healers (supernatural healers) as *daus, chelas*, priest, *lamas,* herbalists and public health practitioners. The Indigenous Health Care System is based on personalistic traditions of folk healers and traditional herbalists. The theoretical side of traditional medical system, the religious backdrop, particularly the belief in the fear of evil spirits, and healing performed according to spiritual rites explains the continuance of indigenous system. The folk healers operate within a religious model, and hence there is no printed or written material to confirm or support the tradition. The indigenous medical system has sustained in society's social cultural complexes through deep rooted processes. It is based on the concepts of health and illness and reflects certain values, traditions and beliefs based on people's way of life.

With changing life styles and introduction of immediate economic return in terms of cash, the traditional values related to the profession of folk healers is changing. The body of indigenous medical knowledge has contributed in the development in health care but with the rapid industrialization, this knowledge is disappearing and needs conservation. People in Himalayan region have a close association with nature. They use psycho-somatic treatment which depends on propitiating the local deities or spirits together with herbal and mineral based medicine. The healers, prescribing these medicines, use vast treasure of indigenous knowledge which needs to be exhaustively explored, revived and used for economic regeneration of mountain communities, as also for the medical benefit of the world at large. Himachal has extensive and deep folk traditions which offer an opportunity and possibility for revival and strengthening of traditional knowledge. The traditional medical system has survived in the region for a very long time, its therapeutic value and what is retainable of this system and how these can be upgraded through education, licensing and incorporation into state health planning still needs to be taken up and linked.

References

Abbink, J. (1995). Medicinal and ritual plants of ethiopia southwest: An account of recent research. *Indigenous Knowledge and Development Monitor, 3*, 6–8.

Anon. (1993). Medicinal plants of Nepal. Bulletin of the Department of Medicinal Plants No. 3. His Majesty's Government of Nepal, Ministry of Forests and Soil Conservation, Department of Medicinal Plants, Thapathali, Kathmandu, Nepal.

Arjariya, A., & Chaurasia, K. (2009). Some medicinal plants among the tribes of Chhatarpur District (M.P.) India. *Ecoprint, 16*, 43–50.

Bhagwan, D. V. (1991). *Materia medica of ayurveda*. New Delhi, India: Jain Publishers.

Bown, D. (1995). *Encyclopaedia of herbs and their uses*. New York: DK Publishing Inc.

Bright, P. S. (2000). India's alternative therapies: The cure of modern times. Junior Science Refresher, pp. 20–27.

Cerqueira, M.T. (2010). Bridging the knowledge-action gap in diabetes along the U.S.-Mexico border. Revista Panamericana de Salud Pública, p. 28.

Dastur, J. F. (1951). *Medicinal plants of India and Pakistan*. Bombay, India: D. B. Taraporevala Sons Co., Ltd.

Ehsan, B. R., Vital, A., & Bipinraj, N. K. (2009). Antimicrobial activity of the ethanolic extract of bryonopsis laciniosa leaf, stem, fruit and seed. *African Journal of Biotechnology, 8*, 3565–3567.

Gupta, V. K., Fatima, A., Faridi, U., et al. (2008). Antimicrobial potential of Glycyrrhiza glabra roots. *Journal of Ethnopharmacology, 116*, 377–380.

International Diabetes Federation (IDF). (2009). The diabetes atlas (4th ed). International Diabetes Federation, Brussels. Retrieved March, 2013 from http://www.diabetesatlas.org/

Jain, A., Choubey, S., Singour, P. K., Rajak, H., & Pawar, R. S. (2011). Sida cordifolia (Linn)—An overview. *Journal of Applied Pharmaceutical Science, 1*, 23–31.

Jain, S.K. (1991). Dictionary of Indian folk medicine and ethno-botany—A reference manual of man—plant relationships, ethnic groups and ethno-botanists in India.

Kamble, S. Y., Patil, S. R., Sawant, P. S., Sawant, S., Pawar, S. G., & Singh, E. A. (2010). Studies on plants used in traditional medicine by Bhilla Tribe of Maharashtra. *Indian Journal of Traditional Knowledge, 9*, 591–598.

Kapahi, B. K., Srivastava, T. N., & Sarin, Y. K. (1993). Description of Picrorhiza kurroa, A Source of Ayurvedic drug Kutaki. *International Journal of Pharmacognosy, 31*(3), 217–222.

Kulkarni, P. H. (2000). *Ayurvedic treatment*. New Delhi, India: Sri Satguru.

Meena, A. K., & Rao, M. M. (2010). Folk herbal medicines used by the Meena community in Rajasthan. *Asian Journal of Traditional Medicines, 5*, 19–31.

Nalini, S. H., & Thomas, W. M. (2009). Review of Glycyrrhiza glabra, Linn. *Siddha Papers, 2*, 1–7.

Negi, J. S., Singh, P., Joshi, G. P., Rawat, M. S., & Bisht, V. K. (2010). Chemical constituents of asparagus. *Pharmacognosy Review, 4*, 215–220.

Ramachandran, A., Snehalatha, C., & Krishnaswamy, C.V. (1995). IDDM registry in India. *Journal of Association* of *Physicians* of *India, 59*, pp. 8–10.

Sharma, R. K., & Dash, V. B. (2002). *Agnivesa's Caraka Samhita: Text with English translation and critical exposition based on Cakrapani Datta's ayurveda dipika*. Varanasi, India: Chowkhamba Sanskrit Series Office.

Shivanna, M. B., & Rajakumar, N. (2010). Ethno-medico-botanical Knowledge of rural folk in Bhadravathi taluk of Shimoga District, Karnataka. *Indian Journal of Traditional Knowledge, 9*, 158–162.

Shukla, R., Chakravarty, M., & Gautam, M. P. (2008). Indigenous medicine used for treatment of gynaecological disorders by tribal of Chhattisgarh, India. *Journal of Medicinal Plants Research, 2*, 356–360.

Tinker, A., Finn, K., & Epp, J. (2000). Improving women's health: Issues and Interventions.HNP Discussion Paper. *The International Bank for Reconstruction and Development, World.*

Tsarong, T. J. (1986). *Handbook of traditional Tibetan drugs: Their nomenclature, composition, use and dosage*. Kalimpong: Tibetan Medical Publications.

Verma, V., Jalalpure, S. S., Sahu, A., Bhardwaj, L. K., & Prakesh, Y. (2011). Bombax ceiba Linn: Pharmacognostical, Phytochemistry, ethnobotany, and pharmacology studies. *Internationale Pharmaceutica Sciencia, 1*, 62–68.

WHO. (2002a). Traditional medicine-growing needs and potential. *WHO Policy Perspectives on Medicine, 2*, 1–6.

WHO. (2002). WHO Traditional Medicine Strategy 2002–2005. Geneva: WHO.

WHO. (2005). *National policy on traditional medicine and regulation of herbal medicines*. Geneva: Report of WHO Global Survey.

WHO. (2009). *Women and health: Today's evidence tomorrow's agenda*. Geneva: WHO Report.

Wild, S., Roglic, G., Green, A., Sicree, R., & King, H. (2004). Global prevalence of diabetes: Estimates for the year 2000 and projections for 2030. *Diabetes Care, 27*, 1047–1053.

Zhang, Y.-J., Li, W., & Zheng, M. (1994). *Chinese-English Chinese traditional medicine world dictionary*. Shanxi, China: Shanxi People's Press.

Chapter 6
Indigenous *Materia Medica*

...The revival interest in herbal medicine is a worldwide phenomenon...

Mark Blumenthal

Abstract Medicinal plants of North-western Himalayas with superb curative properties mentioned in the indigenous *Materia Medica*, are finding application in modern bio-pharmaceuticals. But, due to lack of information regarding the identification, classification and therapeutic values, the knowledge on the value of these is getting reduced. The development of the traditional systems of medicine with the attitude of safety, efficacy and distinction will not only help to safeguard the traditional legacy of Himalayas but also to streamline the utilization of natural products in the health care.

Keywords *Materia Medica* · Medicinal plants · Traditional system of medicine · Traditional medicinal formulations · Therapeutic value · Salts and minerals

The Indian *Materia Medica* contains nearly 2,000 drugs, the majority of which are of plant origin. At the time of Great king *Ashoka* in Hindu *Materia Medica* one finds the mention of nearly 700 herbal medicines. The student of medicine used to learn the art of healing by living with the *Guru* in the *Gurukulas* who use to impart the practical training to the student with regard to identification, collection and utilization of medicinal plants. With the passage of time more and more medicinal plants were included in the *Materia Medica*. In the following section the descriptive account of herbs and other curative substances used by herbalists across the North-western Himalayas is presented. The *Materia Medica* of Himalayan Medicines is considerable when compared to other indigenous systems of medicine in India. It involves the usage of herbal products, like plant bark, resin, leaves, root, rhizome, stem, etc. besides, minerals and chemicals obtained from natural form. The *Ayurvedic* study of medicinal herbs is called *Dravya-guna-karma Vigyana*, which exactly means the science of material, their qualities and actions. Material substances include both food and herbs. Each plant and its parts are believed to possess the life-giving essence. Thus, *Materia Medica* is basically a synthesis of information on herbal and non-herbal drugs, their gathering, method

P. Gupta et al., *Healing Traditions of the Northwestern Himalayas*,
SpringerBriefs in Environmental Science, DOI: 10.1007/978-81-322-1925-5_6,

of acquiring, handing and administration in the traditional health care systems. In the context of wearing away indigenous knowledge base, this endeavour is very essential and hence an effort has been made to make to prepare a *Materia Medica* of North-western Himalayas. There is need of blending the folk wisdom with the contemporary scientific knowledge, which can be possible only when the scientific community recognises and makes use of the best of the folk medical practices. For this purpose, the scientists must have an association with the folk-healers, where learning from their experiences and scientifically validation can provide impetus to the modern medicine. In turn, the efforts of folk practitioners must be acknowledged, which will certainly provide them a reputable place in the society. The interactive sessions and workshops for the scientific community and folk healers will provide a platform for both and will be equally benefit the two.

6.1 Material Used by Folk Herbalists

6.1.1 Medicinal Plants

A number of medicinal plants are used by the herbalists for preparing medicines. Some of them are *Abrus precatorius, Aconitum deinorrhizum, Aconitum heterophylum, Acorus calamus, Aegle marmelos, Ajuga bracteosa, Albizia lebbeck, Aloe barbadensis, Arnebia sp. Asparagus abscendens, Azadirachata indica, Bauhinia variegate, Berberis aristata, Bergenia ciliate, Betula utilis, Bombax ceiba, Butea monosperma, Calotropis gigantean, Cassia fistula, Cedrus deodara, Cichorium intybus, Cinnamomum tamala, Cissampelos pareira, Acacia catechu, Magnifera indica, Zingiber officinale, Trachyspermum ammi, Cuscuta reflexa, Juglans regia, Linum usitatissimum, Solanum tuberosum, Spondias pinnata, Emblica officinalis, Ricinus communis, Prunus persica, Bambusa sp., Vitex negundo, Ficus bengalensis, Aegle marmelos, Zizyphus jujube, Cannabis sativa, Grevia oppositifolia, Girardinia hetrophylla, Swertia chirayita, Euphorbia royleana, Punica granatum, Oryza sativa, Coriandrum sativum, Datura metel, Cynodon dactylon, Murraya koenigii, Calendula officinalis, Citrus limon, Morchella sp., Rosa sp., Tinospora cordifolia, Curcuma langa, Syzium cumini, Hordeum vulgare, Bunium persicum, Gentiana kurroo, Pistacia intergerrima, Momordica charantia, Indigofera gerradiana, Aloe barbadensis, Allium sativum, Trigonella foenum, Ficus religiosa, Fumaria officinalis, Allium cepa, Mentha viridus, Achyranthes aspera, Agave Americana, Sapindus mukorossi, Vinca rosea, Eucalyptus globules, Brassica juncea, Bombax ceiba, Dalbergia sissoo, Bauhinia vahlii, Sesamum indicum, Ocimum sanctum, Zanthoxylum armatum, Swertia chirayita, Operculina turpethum, Carissa carandus, Clerodendrum serratum, Corydalis govaniana, Crocus sativus, Cuscuta reflexa, Cyperus rotundus, Dactylorhiza hatagirea, Fagopyrum esculentum, Gentiana kurroo, Hedychium acuminatum*, etc. Some of the plants are available locally, while others are procured from outside the state.

The history of sale of raw drug in Himachal is less than a 100 years old. There are numerous rare manuscripts which describe the causes and cures of various diseases. These are usually lying in the custody of priests or *lamas*. In district *Kinnaur* these manuscripts are known as *Pothies* whereas in district Shimla these are popularly known as *Sancha granth*. The *Pothies* are usually written in Tibetan language and contain information on the cause and remedy of various diseases. These manuscripts contain information on method of preparation of drugs, dosage and precautions. The *Pothies* usually consists of loose sheets of birch bark on which the information is written. Some of these are hand written whereas some others prepared by using traditional block printing technique. Information on the detailed description of plant/animal, etc., used in the preparation of drugs is given in these. The methods of diagnosis and treatment including spiritual healing and therapeutic procedures are described in the *pothies*. *Sancha,* on the other hand carries information pertaining to influence of planets on the health and general well-being of the person. These contain astrological and numerological calculations on festive occasions, good and bad time and occurrence of solar and lunar eclipses. *Sancha* is written in *Tankri* script. Specific days are marked for writing these manuscripts. While using *Sancha,* the user, who is an expert in interpretation, uses a dice. The dice is tossed and the calculations are made. The interpretation of calculations is read from the manuscript. This helps in finding the cause and cure of problems. Once the cause of problem is explored, the next step is finding the solution. These manuscripts are kept in a temple or at sanctified place. *Sancha* also carries information on various procedures which are used for resolving health problems. The tradition of conventional healing can be traced back to several centuries. Therefore, it can be presumed that a market for these medicines must have existed for years. Nearly 70 % of the plants and other material used in the formulations are locally available and 30 % is procured from outside. Erosion of knowledge on the availability of raw material used for the preparation of medicines is the reason for fading of health traditions. Initially, the job of collecting raw material and formulation preparation was confined to the family members of healers, which was done under the supervision and advice of the elders. The elders provided the list of raw material, quantity to be used and mode of preparation of herbal formulations. Some locals who use to collect medicinal plants were also engaged to procure rare and hard-to get plants. Thus, the drugs pass through the hands of local collectors and traders before reaching the end user. However, due to the erosion of knowledge-base, it is becoming difficult to procure and prepare medicines without seeking the help of knowledgeable beings. Some of the locally non-available raw material is brought to the market from neighbouring states of Himachal Pradesh (Table 6.1).

Table 6.1 *Materia Medica* of traditional system of medicine (Appendices A–C)

#	Scientific name of plant	Vernacular name	Part used	Therapeutic value
1.	*Abrus precatorius* Linn.	Ratti/chuntli	Leaves	Act as purgative and abortifacient
2.	*Acacia catechu* Linn.	Khair	Bark	Used for treating mouth sores and cancer
3.	*Acacia concinna* Willd.	Shikakai	Pods	Pods used for washing hair. Effective in scalp treatment
4.	*Acacia nilotica* Willd.	Kikar	Flower, pod	Leaves effective in sore throat and sore eyes. Stem used for cleaning teeth
5.	*Achyranthes aspera* Linn.	Puthkanda	Stem, root, leaf, seeds	Seeds act as antidote to snake poison, leaf paste is applied on scorpion stings. Plant ash cures dropsy and root act as abortifacient
6.	*Aconitium heterophyllum* Wall.	Atish/patish	Whole plant	Utilized in the preparation meant for the gastrointestinal disorders
7.	*Aconitum deinorrhizum Stapf.*	Vatsnabh	Tubers	Used in the medicinal formulations
8.	*Acorus calamus* Linn.	Barjay	Rhizome	Leaves used for treating Bronchitis. Leaf paste is applied on nose and throat
9.	*Aegle marmelos* Linn.	Bel	Leaves, fruits	Fruits are effective in diarrhoea and dysentery
10.	*Agave americana* Linn.	Ramban	Stem	Stalk cooked as vegetable and cures digestive disorders. Plant extract is dropped in ear to cure ear ache
11.	*Ajuga bracteosa* Linn.	Neelkanthi	Leaves	Effectively cures fever and controls diabetes
12.	*Albizia lebbeck* (L.) Benth.	Siris/kala siris	Bark, leaves, flowers	Treats cough and cold. Flower paste is used for curing boils/swelling. Act as antidote to poisons. Powdered bark is effective in treating ulcers
13.	*Allium cepa* Linn.	Piyaz	Bulb	Bulb juice is administrated in dyspepsia and sun strokes
14.	*Allium sativum* Linn.	Lahasun	Scale leaves	Control gastric problems and effective in arthritis
15.	*Aloe barbadensis* (L.) Burm.	Kawarpatha	Stem	Possess anti-diabetic properties and its extract is a best remedy for hair fall and dandruff
16.	*Anacyclus Pyrethrum* (L.) Link	Akarkara	Flower	Effective in dental problems
17.	*Anethum graveolens* Linn.	Kadvi saunf	Seeds	Effective in dysentery
18.	*Anogeissus latifolia* Roxb. Ex DC.	Dhav	Leaves, bark	Gynaecological problems
19.	*Apium graveolens* Mill.	Ajmod	Fruit	Effective in digestive and hepatobiliary disorders
20.	*Arnebia* sp.	Ratanjot	Roots	Effective in treating burns, scalp problems and dandruff
21.	*Artemesia* sp.	Kayankaya	Leaves	Fresh stem is consumed in dried form and given to livestock

(continued)

Table 6.1 (continued)

#	Scientific name of plant	Vernacular name	Part used	Therapeutic value
22.	*Asparagus racemosus* Willd.	Kelti	Roots	Used for controlling dysentery and in the preparation of traditional medicinal formulations
23.	*Azadirachta indica* Linn.	Neem	Whole plant	Useful in diabetes and skin problems
24.	*Bambusa* sp.	Baans	Stem	Used for preparing *banslochan*
25.	*Bauhinia vahlii* Wight and Arnott	Taur	Latex	Latex is used for curing acne
26.	*Bauhinia variegata* Linn.	Kachnar	Roots, bark, buds	Useful in controlling dysentery
27.	*Berberis aristata* Linn.	Kashmal	Roots	Roots utilized for extracting *rasont* which is used in traditional formulations meant for curing eye problems.
28.	*Bergenia ciliate* Haw.	Phorach/ Pashanbheda	Leaf, root	Act as diuretic
29.	*Betula utilis* Wall.	Bhojpatra	Bark	Paste is used for expelling placenta in livestock
30.	*Bombax ceiba* Linn.	Semal	Roots, bark, flowers, fruits	Consumption of flower bud treats leucorrhoea. Effective in gastric problem, toothache/mouth ulcers
31.	*Brassica juncea* Linn.	Sarson	Seeds	Effective for digestive disorders
32.	*Bryonopsis laciniosa* Linn.	Shivlingi	Seeds	Gynaecological problems
33.	*Bunium persicum* Boiss.	Kala zeera	Seeds	Useful in treating digestive and gynaecological problems
34.	*Butea monosperma* Lam.	Palas	Flower, seeds, leaves	Regulate menstrual flow and act as abortifacient
35.	*Calendula officinalis* Linn.	Gainda	Flowers	Flower paste is used for treating piles
36.	*Calotropis gigantea* Linn.	Aak	Leaves, latex	Extract of roots and leaves has anticancer properties and is effective in curing wounds. Its latex is used for treating tooth ache
37.	*Cannabis sativa* Linn.	Bhang	Leaves, seeds	Leaf extract is good remedy for insect bite
38.	*Capsicumannuum* Linn.	Lal mirch	Fruit	Useful in treating Mumps
39.	*Carica papaya* Linn.	Papita	Fruit	Fruit given to diabetic patient. Roots of the plant are used for preparing eye medicine. Root extract is put in eyes. Unripe fruit acts as abortifacient
40.	*Carissa carandas* Linn.	Karonda	Fruits	Used in the preparation of medicines

(continued)

Table 6.1 (continued)

#	Scientific name of plant	Vernacular name	Part used	Therapeutic value
41.	*Cassia angustifolia* M. Vahl	Sanaya	Stem	Effective in gastrointestinal disorders
42.	*Cassia fistula* Linn.	Amaltas	Leaves, root, pod	Used for treating gastrointestinal disorders
43.	*Cedrus deodara* Roxb.	Deodar	Stem	Resin used in formulations, wood as splinter in bone fracture
44.	*Chlorophytum borivilianum* Linn.	Safedmusli	Root	Tonic useful in handling gynaecological problems
45.	*Cicer arietinum* Linn.	Channa	Seeds	Skin disorders
46.	*Cichorium intybus* Linn.	Kasani butti	Roots	Effectively cures fever and vomiting
47.	*Cinnamomum tamala* Buch.-Ham.	Tejpatta	Leaf	Effective in diarrhoea/colic pain.
48.	*Cinnamomum zeylanicum* Breyn.	Kuranday/ kurundu	Fruits	Thorns are used to take out pus from the wound. Latex is effective in treating wounds
49.	*Cissampelos pareira* Linn.	Patindu	Leaves, stem, root	Act as antidote to poison
50.	*Citrus limon* Burm.	Galgal	Leaves, fruits	Leaves are tied on abdomen for stomach-ache
51.	*Clerodendrum serratum* Linn.	Banbakri	Roots, leaves	Leaf paste is effective in treating herpes eruptions. The paste applied on affected area along with clarified butter
52.	*Coleus amboinicus* Lour.	Pashanbedh	Leaves, roots	Effective in Urinary problems
53.	*Commiphora guggul* (Arn.) Bhandari	Gugal	Gum	Act as antispasmodic, effective in rheumatic pains
54.	*Coriandrum sativum* Linn.	Dhania	Leaves, seeds	Used for treating digestive disorders and eye problems
55.	*Corydalis govaniana* Wall.	Bhutkesi	Roots	Used as a diuretic
56.	*Crocus sativus* Linn.	Kesar	Stigma	Act as nervous tonic
57.	*Cucumis melo* Linn.	Kheera	Fruit	Fruit extract cures burning micturition
58.	*Cucurbita argyrosperma* K. Koch	Kadu	Whole plant	Useful in gastrointestinal problems
59.	*Cuminum cyminum* Linn.	Zeera	Seeds	Curing digestive disorders
60.	*Curcuma longa* Linn.	Haldi	Rhizome	Its paste prepared in mustard oil is effective in wound healing. Extract cures gum problems
61.	*Curcuma zedoaria* Linn.	Kachur	Fruit, rhizome	Effective in stomach-ache, leucoderma
62.	*Cuscuta reflexa* Roxb.	Akashbael	Stem, leaves	Used in number of formulations meant for gastrointestinal disorders also effective in skin disorders

(continued)

Table 6.1 (continued)

#	Scientific name of plant	Vernacular name	Part used	Therapeutic value
63.	*Cynodon dactylon* Linn.	Dhruv	Whole plant	Used in the preparation of medicines. Act as diuretic
64.	*Cyperus rotundus* Linn.	Nagarmotha	Root	Effective in diarrhoea and wounds healing. Root extract is anti-inflammatory
65.	*Dactylorhiza hatagirea* D. Don	Salamepanjaa	Roots	Act as a tonic, also effective in fever
66.	*Datura metel* Linn.	Dhatura	Leaves, fruits	Leaves are used for treating stomach ache. Clarified butter is applied on leaves and tied on the stomach. Application of leaf paste of *Ocimum sanctum, Ficus religiosa* and *Datura metel* is effective in inflammation
67.	*Delphinium denudatum* Wall.	Narbishi	Leaves	Effective in ear-ache
68.	*Dioscorea deltoidea* Wall. ex Kunth	Singli mingli	Rhizome	Effective in allergies and rheumatic diseases
69.	*Dolichos biflorus* Linn.	Kulth	Whole plant	Used for treating urinary problems
70.	*Elettaria cardamomum* Linn.	Elayache	Fruit, seeds	Curing digestive disorders, cough and cold
71.	*Emblica officinalis* Gaertn.	Amla	Fruit	Used formulations meant for gastrointestinal disorders
72.	*Ephedra gerardiana* Linn.	Chee	Shoot	Beneficial in the bronchitis asthma and allergy
73.	*Eucalyptus globulus* Labill.	Safeda	Leaves	Cures cough and cold
74.	*Euphorbia hirta* Linn.	Dudhli	Latex	Effective in skin disorders
75.	*Euphorbia royleana* Boiss.	Churro	Stem	Latex is used for curing digestive disorders and insect bite
76.	*Fagopyrum esculentum* Moench.	Ogla	Fruit	Helpful in pain and inflammation
77.	*Ficus carica* Linn.	Anjeer	Fruit	Helpful in worm infestation
78.	*Ficus religiosa* Linn.	Pipal	Leaf, bark	Fruits of trees are used for medicinal purpose of infants
79.	*Fumariaparviflora* Linn.	Pithpapara	Leaves	Reduces blood pressure, used for treating skin problems
80.	*Gentiana kurroo* Royle	Karu	Rhizome	Effective in treating diabetes, fever and inflammation. Used as a blood purifier, Anthelmintic and tonic
81.	*Girardinia heterophylla* Link.	Bichubutti	Leaves	Leaf paste is effective in paralysis and stoke
82.	*Glycerrhiza glabra* Linn.	Mulethi	Fruit	Cough and cold
83.	*Grewia oppositifolia* Linn.	Bheul	Leaves, stem	Used for preparing medicines (eruption, fever, bone fracture as splinter)
84.	*Gymnema sylvestre* R. Br.	Gudmaar	Leaves	Effective in diabetes

(continued)

Table 6.1 (continued)

#	Scientific name of plant	Vernacular name	Part used	Therapeutic value
85.	*Hedychium acuminatum* Wall.	Kachur	Rhizome	Effective in digestive disorders, aches and inflammations
86.	*Hippophae rhamnoides* Linn.	Chharma	Fruits	Used in medicines and cosmetics
87.	*Holarrhena antidysenterica* Wall.	Indrajau	Seeds	Effective for treating diarrhoea and worm infestation
88.	*Hordeum vulgare* Linn.	Jau	Seeds and grass	For preparing *Jaukshaar*, used in medicinal formulations
89.	*Hyoscyamus niger* Linn.	Tukhlang/ thuklang	Leaves, seeds	Sedative
90.	*Hyssopus officinalis* Linn.	Zuffa	Leaves	Effective in toothache, inflammations, and throat sores
91.	*Indigofera gerardiana* Wall. Ex Baker.	Kathi	Leaves	It is good for digestive disorders and act as Anthelmintic
92.	*Ipomoea digitata* Linn.	Vidarikand	Rhizome	Used as aphrodisiac. Useful in soreness of cough, act as diuretic
93.	*Juglans regia* Linn.	Akhrot	Bark, fruit	Bark used for cleansing teeth
94.	*Juniperus communis* Linn.	Dhaamaa/ Hapusha/ theleru/ chhershup/	Berry, bark, needles	Urinary tract disinfectant, effective in curing asthma, act as a diuretic and cures leucorrhoea
95.	*Jurinea dolomiaea* Boiss.	Dhoop	Roots	Effective in skin eruptions and oil cures body aches
96.	*Justicia adhatoda* Linn.	Bainchtay/Basuti/ Nirgandi	Leaves, roots	Leaf extract is used for curing acne, which is applied on the skin with mustard oil. The same extract is effective in *Pityriasis capitis*. *Chui* (a traditional shampoo) is prepared by boiling its leaves in water. Root act as Abortifacient
97.	*Lawsonia inermis* Linn.	Mehandi	Leaves	Skin problems
98.	*Lens esculenta* Moench.	Masur	Seeds	Effective in skin problems
99.	*Linum usitatissimum* Linn.	Alsi	Seeds	Poultice of seeds is used for curing acne. Seeds used in number of formulations
100.	*Mangifera indica* Linn.	Aam	Bark, leaf fruit	Used in the preparation of medicines for treating diabetes
101.	*Medicago falcata* Linn.	Kuthae	Leaves	Highly nutritive

(continued)

Table 6.1 (continued)

#	Scientific name of plant	Vernacular name	Part used	Therapeutic value
102.	*Mentha longifolia* Linn.	Koshu	Leaves	Cures nausea
103.	*Mentha viridis* Linn.	Podina	Leaves	Cures dyspepsia
104.	*Mesua ferrea* Linn.	Nagkesar	Stamens, fruits	Effective in diarrhoea, leucorrhoea and bleeding piles
105.	*Momordica charantia* Descourt.	Karela	Fruits	Helpful in controlling diabetes
106.	*Morchella esculenta* Linn.	Guchhi	Whole body	Paste as household remedy for burns
107.	*Mucuna pruriens* Linn.	Kauch	Seeds	Effective in infertility
108.	*Murraya koenigii* Linn.	Gadhela	Leaves	Leaves considered good for heart problems. Stem used for cleaning teeth
109.	*Musa paradisiaca* Linn.	Kela	Fruit, root	Unripe fruit is effective for diabetes. Root extract cures burning of eyes
110.	*Myrica nagi* Thunb.	Kaiphal	Fruits, bark	Fruit effective in diarrhoea. Bark is chewed for tooth-ache
111.	*Myristica fragrans* Houtt.	Jayfal	Fruit	Used in various medicinal formulation. Fruit's paste, if applied locally, is effective remedy for acne and if fed orally treats stomach ache
112.	*Myrsine africana* Linn.	Baibidang	Fruit	For treating worm infestation, colic and blood purification
113.	*Nardostachys grandiflora* D. Don.	Jatamansi	Rhizome	Act as anti-spasmodic, hair tonic and heart tonic
114.	*Nelumbonucifera* Gaertn.	Tal makhana	Fruit	It boosts energy, stamina and vitality. Effective in jaundice, arthritis and rheumatism
115.	*Nerium indicum* Mill.	Kaner	Leaves, flowers	Effective in skin diseases
116.	*Ocimum sanctum* Linn.	Tulsi	Leaf	Plant is herbal remedy for common body ailments. Leaf juice is given to cure fever, dysentery and dyspepsia
117.	*Operculina turpethum* Linn.	Nishoth	Leaves	Cures digestive disorders
118.	*Origanum vulgare* Linn.	Jakhm-buti	Leaves	Useful in wound healing and skin diseases
119.	*Oryza sativa* Linn.	Dhaan	Seeds	Cooked rice tied around throat for treating mumps (*Epidemic parotitis*). Rice water is given to treat dysentery
120.	*Oxyria* sp.	Surchee	Whole plant	Cures dyspepsia
121.	*Pandanus odoratissimus* Linn.	Kewda	Flower	Effective in diabetes
122.	*Papaversomniferum* Linn.	Afimdana	Seeds	Treats digestive disorders
123.	*Phoenix sylvestris* (L.) Roxb.	Khajur	Leaves, fruits	Cures digestive problems
124.	*Picrorhiza kurroa* Royle ex Benth	Kutki/karru	Rhizome	Effective in digestive disorders, bronchial asthma

(continued)

Table 6.1 (continued)

#	Scientific name of plant	Vernacular name	Part used	Therapeutic value
125.	*Pinus roxburghii* Roxb.	Chir	Stem, needles	Oil utilized in medicines, wood as splinter in fracture
126.	*Pinus wallichiana* A. B. Jacks	Kail	Resin	Effectively heals cuts and wounds, wood used as splinter for bone fractures
127.	*Piper longum* Linn.	Mugh	Root	Effective in cough and cold
128.	*Piper nigrum* Linn.	Kalimirch	Seeds	Treats bronchitis and skin disorders
129.	*Pistacia integerrima*J.L.Stewart	Kakarsinghi	Stem	Dried stem is burnt and ash mixed with honey relieves cough and cold
130.	*Plantago ovata* Forssk.	Isabogol	Seeds	Effective in digestive disorders
131.	*Poa cynosuroides* Linn.	Kusha	Runner	Cure dysentery and urinary disorders
132.	*Podophyllum hexandrum* Royle	Bankakri	Rhizome	Effective in worm infestation and cutaneous diseases
133.	*Prinsepia utilis* Royle	Bhekhal	Kernel oil	Oil used for treating *rheumatic* diseases
134.	*Prunella vulgaris* Linn.	Khadus	Leaves	Cures mouth ulcers, wounds and cuts
135.	*Prunus armeniaca* Linn.	Chulli	Fruit, kennel oil	Fruit used as laxative, kennel oil for arthritis, ear ache, etc.
136.	*Prunus cerasoides* D. Don.	Pajja	Stem	Cures cough and cold
137.	*Prunus dulcis* Batsch.	Badam	Fruit, seeds	Used in Skin disorders and possess high nutritive value
138.	*Prunus persica* Linn.	Aru	Leaves	Leaf extract is applied on acne or itching skin
139.	*Psoralea corylifolia* Linn.	Babchi	Leaves	Effective for skin diseases
140.	*Punica granatum* Linn.	Daru	Seeds	Seeds used for preparing numerous medicines
141.	*Quercus infectoria* Olivier.	Majuphal	Gall, fruits	Effective for gynaecological problems
142.	*Raphanus sativus* Linn.	Mulli	Root	Root cures jaundice, piles and urinary problems
143.	*Rauwolfia serpentine* Linn.	Sarpgandha	Roots	Used in the treatment of Blood pressure. Plant decoction induces labor pain
144.	*Rheum* sp. Linn.	Arch/Chukri/ Revanchini	Roots	Root extract effective in sprains
145.	*Rhododendron anthopogon* D. Don	Chau	Leaves, flowers	Oil used for rheumatic conditions, affects bones and nervous system
146.	*Rhododendron campanulatum* D. Don	Sermadang	Leaves	Grinded and applied on affected area on itching skin
147.	*Ricinus communis* Linn.	Arind	Seeds, leaves	Leaves used for treating stomach-ache, clarified butter is applied on the leaves and tied on the stomach

(continued)

Table 6.1 (continued)

#	Scientific name of plant	Vernacular name	Part used	Therapeutic value
148.	*Rosa* sp. Linn.	Gulab	Flower	Used in formulations
149.	*Roscoea alpine Royle.*	Safed-musli	Tuber	Tonic for impotency
150.	*Rumex* Linn.	Shoma	Root	Grinded and extract for swelling
151.	*Sapindus mukorossi* Linn.	Reetha	Fruits	It is poisonous. Leaves are used for preparing *choi*, a conventional hair shampoo
152.	*Saussurea costus* Falc.	Kuth	Roots	Cures bronchitis diarrhoea, regulate menstrual disorders
153.	*Scilla indica* Baker.	Jangli piyaz	Bulbs	Effective in worm infestation and digestive disorders. Used in formulation for asthmatic condition
154.	*Semecarpus anacardium* Linn.	Bhallathak	Seeds	Useful in treating scalp conditions
155.	*Sesamum indicum* Linn.	Til	Seeds	Oil is effective in rheumatic pains
156.	*Sida cordifolia* Linn.	Dhreed	Fruit	Effective for gynaecological problems
157.	*Silene cucubalus* Linn.	Murchichee	Whole plant	Nutritious plant
158.	*Solanum tuberosum* Linn.	Alu	Tuber	Used for treating boils and burns
159.	*Solanum xanthocarpum* Schrad. and Wendl.	Kantkari	Root, berries	Used in the preparation of medicines
160.	*Sphaeranthus indicus* Linn.	Gorakmundi	Fruit	Effective in treating piles
161.	*Spilanthes acmella* Linn.	Akarkara	Leaves, flowers	For treating toothache, bleeding gums
162.	*Spondias pinnata* Linn.	Amber	Roots	Utilized in the preparation of numerous formulations
163.	*Swertia chirayita* Roxb.	Chirayata	Leaves	Leaves are given to diabetic patient
164.	*Symplocos crataegoides* DDon.	Lodh	Bark	Used for treatment of ulcers, tumours and eye diseases
165.	*Syzygium aromaticum* Linn.	Lavang	Buds	Effective in gastrointestinal, fever, cough and cold
166.	*Syzygium cumini* Linn.	Jamun	Fruits, leaves	Used in the treatment of diabetes and bronchitis
167.	*Taxus baccata* Linn.	Thangi/rakhala	Needles	Controls cold and headache
168.	*Terminalia arjuna* Roxb.	Arjun	Bark	Employed for treating burns and boils and in the preparation meant for gynaecological disorders
169.	*Terminalia bellirica* Roxb.	Behera	Fruits	Used in the treatment of gastrointestinal and skin disorders

(continued)

Table 6.1 (continued)

#	Scientific name of plant	Vernacular name	Part used	Therapeutic value
170.	*Terminalia chebula* Retz.	Harad	Fruits	Used for preparing medicines meant for digestive and skin disorders.
171.	*Thevetia nerifolia* Pers.	Khanera	Leaves, flowers	Used in the preparation of medicinal formulations
172.	*Thymus serpyllum* Linn.	Banajwain/ Piplichee	Whole plant	Utilized for treating skin diseases, cough and cold
173.	*Tinospora cordifolia* Thumb.	Guljay/Geloyae	Leaves, stem	Used for regulating flow of urine and burning micturition in cattle and human beings. Leaf and stem extract effective in diabetes, digestive disorders and arthritis
174.	*Trachyspermum ammi* Linn.	Ajwain	Seeds	Used for treating gastrointestinal disorders
175.	*Tribulus terrestris* Linn.	Gokhru	Fruit	Effective in arthritis and as an aphrodisiac
176.	*Trigonella foenum* Linn.	Methi	Leaves, seeds	Cures digestive disorders and joint pains. Also effective in diabetes
177.	*Triticum aestivum* Linn.	Ghenu	Seeds	Used in medicinal formulations
178.	*Urtica* sp.	Korgaya	Leaves	Considered 'hot' and consumed for joint pains
179.	*Valeriana wallichii* DC.	Jatamassi	Rhizome	Effective in gastrointestinal disorders
180.	*Vinca rosea*Linn.	Sadabahar	Leaves	Effective in diabetes
181.	*Viola serpens* Wall.	Banaksha	Flowers	Dried flowers are used for preparing decoction effective for cough and cold
182.	*Vitex negundo* Linn.	Banna	Stem, leaves	Leaf extract is effective in acne. Stem used for cleansing teeth. Leaf paste is useful in joint inflammations. Leaves boiled in water used for hot water fomentation relieving pain/sprains
183.	*Withania somnifera* Linn.	Ashvangadha	Leaves	Relieves body aches
184.	*Zanthoxylum armatum* Linn.	Tung/tirmir	Stem, leaves	Effective for bleeding gums, acts as astringent.
185.	*Zea mays* Linn.	Kukari/makki	Seeds and corn silk	Used for the treatment of urinary problems
186.	*Zingiber officinale* Rosc.	Adrak	Rhizome	Extract of rhizome mixed with honey cures cold and cough. Dried rhizome is used for preparing powder, which is cooked and given to women after delivery. Its powder is used in number of decoctions
187.	*Zizyphus jujube* Mill.	Ber	Fruit	Powder of dried seeds is recommended with cumin seeds for relief from nausea and emesis

Table 6.2 Therapeutic utilization of animal/animal parts

#	Vernacular name of the animal	Scientific name of animal	Part used	Therapeutic value
1.	Beer	*Ursus sp.*	Subcutaneous body fat	Fat is applied on affected areas in case of musculoskeletal disorders
2.	Cow	*Bos taurus*	Cow dung	Ash of cow dung cakes mixed with mustard oil if applied on the affected area treats worm infestation Ash of cow dung cakes if applied on infected gums, helps in the removal of infected blood
3.	Goat	*Capra hircus*	Subcutaneous body fat	Effective in musculoskeletal disorders
4.	Horse	*Equus caballus*	Faecal matter	In the preparation of Tibetan medicine
5.	Jackal	*Cannis sp.*	Subcutaneous body fat	Fat is boiled/heated and applied on affected areas for treating musculoskeletal disorders
6.	Kumardi	*Polyspis sp.*	Mud produced by the insect	Mud mixed in honey is orally administered for treating dyspepsia
7.	Mangan	*Cimex sp.*	Whole insect	In the preparation of medicinal formulations
8.	Peacock	*Pavo cristatus*	Feather	Ash of peacock feather mixed with honey is effective in treating dyspepsia
9.	Pig	*Sus domesticus*	Faecal matter	In the preparation of Tibetan medicine
10.	Raal	*Nemorhaedus goral*	Horn	For treating rheumatic pains
11.	Riungal	*Vespa sp.*	Poison	Sting poison is used for treating rheumatic pains
12.	Sheep	*Ovis aries*	Milk	Unboiled milk is effective in mouth ulcers

6.1.2 Animal/Animal parts

Animal body parts, for instance, bones, feathers, faecal matter, hair, fat, milk, etc. are used in traditional medicinal formulations. Some of the animals having ethnozoological significance are (Table 6.2).

6.1.3 Minerals/Salts

Along with plants and animal matter, a few salts and minerals are also used in medicinal formulations. A few among these are (Table 6.3).

Table 6.3 Therapeutic utilization of minerals

Sr. No.	Common name of mineral/salt	Scientific/ English name	Therapeutic value
1.	Chunna	Lime	Mixed in water, if applied on boils and burns cures the same
2.	Fitkari	Alum	Effective in cuts and wounds
3.	Gandhak	Sulphur	In the preparation of conventional medicinal formulations
4.	Geru	Red clay	In the preparation of conventional medicinal formulations
5.	Hing	Ferula asafoetida	Used in the treatment of cough and cold, digestive disorders
6.	Kala namak	Saltpetre	Effective in the treatment of digestive disorders
7.	Kapoor	*Cinnamomum camphone*	In the preparation of conventional medicinal formulations
8.	Nausader	Chloride of ammonia	In the preparation of conventional medicinal formulations especially those meant for urinary problems
9.	Neela thotha	Copper sulphate	Effective in treating mouth ulcers
10.	Para	Mercury	In the preparation of conventional medicinal formulations
11.	Sangraph	Ore of mercury	Used in the number of medicinal formulations
12.	Suhaga	Borax powder	Treatment of mouth ulcers
13.	Zeharmohara	Serpentine stone	Effective in treating snakebite
14.	Shilajit	Asphaltum/ Ozokerite	Improves stamina, relieves stress and effective in musculoskeletal disorders

Medicinal plants available in the North-western Himalayas have wonderful curative properties and are finding application in modern bio-pharmaceuticals. But, due to lack of knowledge of identification, classification and therapeutic values, the knowledge on the value of these is getting diminished. Taking benefit of tribal and rural folks, the traders procure valuable herbs without revealing their real value, at a very low price and sell these in markets at a quite high price. Cultivation of important medicinal plants and conservation of wild herbs, if undertaken scientifically, will pave the way for expansion of medicinal plant sector in the near future. The region will have higher livelihood options, if the dissemination of the knowledge of traditional knowledge on medicinal plants is done properly.

Herbal medicine is once again viewed for the management of health problems. Numerous modern drugs are derived from prototypic molecules in medicinal herbs. The traditional medicines in use are derived from vegetal, minerals and organic matter. The traditional knowledge with its holistic approach supported by long-established trial base can serve as an inventive and influential discovery engine for latest, secure and reasonable medicines. The plant species mentioned in the traditional healing systems must be explored with the contemporary scientific approaches for making improvements in health care sector. The development of the traditional systems of medicine with the attitude of security, effectiveness and excellence will not only help to safeguard the traditional legacy of Himalayas but also to rationalize the utilization of natural products in the health care.

Epilogue

...Written words in solitary are medicine....
Sharon Greatwood Callen

Traditional wisdom grew as a result of close interdependence between knowledge, geographical and socio-cultural milieu of aboriginal societies and its oral propagation in accordance with cultural principles. Rules regarding its privacy and inviolability governed the management of these systems. Maintaining good health by employing folk therapeutic procedures and utilization of herbs is as old as the history of humanity. Traditional health care systems have evolved even much before the development of modern medicine. Today, the world is looking back at the alternative system of medicine, because it strives to investigate and cure the cause of a disease, covering up all its symptoms. In the recent years, the use of the alternative system of medicine has got wide attention and recognition throughout the world. In some Asian and African countries, 80 % of the population depend on the traditional medicine for primary health care. It considers each one as a sole individual and is a holistic approach of treatment. The alternative medicine makes use of time-tested natural remedies and is hands-on treatment. The knowledge on conventional healing techniques, which still exists in the form of unrecorded *materia medica* of Himalayan communities is slowly fading away and traditions linked with passing on of traditional wisdom from one generation to another is dilapidating. The significance of safeguarding indigenous medical knowledge in the context of cultural milieu of the Himalayan region is becoming critical. This book has focused at customary folk healing traditions of the North-Western Himalayas. Besides, gathering people's perception of disease, concept of healing, and evolution of folk medicine, an attempt has been made to illustrate diverse therapeutic procedures adopted by folk healers and their implications in the socio-cultural life of Himalayan societies.

Traditional medicines rely exclusively on practical experiences and observation handed down from one generation to another. In the contemporary world, medical treatment is done by allopathic medicine and surgery, which although cures quickly but leaves its scares in the body, while alternate system of medicine addresses larger discourse. It believes in gentle, long-term support to facilitate

P. Gupta et al., *Healing Traditions of the Northwestern Himalayas*,
SpringerBriefs in Environmental Science, DOI: 10.1007/978-81-322-1925-5,

body's own innate powers to heal. Mountain communities have inherited a variety of traditions, dialects and beliefs and have ways to make use of natural resources around them in numerous ways. The use of minerals, plants, animals, etc., for treating diseases is very common, and has paved way for the progression of traditional system of healing.

The indigenous medical systems are still prevalent in the Himalayan region because of their aptness, ease of access and appreciation, which encourage communities to make use of these systems for meeting the health care needs. Still, a number of gaps exist with regard to the limitations and prospects of traditional medicine. Understanding the insight of folk healers and relationship between spiritual and folk healing is also lacking. Today's changing environmental and socio-economic scenario is posing threats not only to herbal wealth but also to ethno-botanical wisdom of its custodians, which is on the verge of extinction. The approaches on preservation and sustainable use of herbs are yet unusual. And with the passage of time, the wisdom associated with healing, if not documented, will fade into oblivion, hence call for preservation.

Traditional healing takes into account the psychological and social aspects of a problem. No matter what are the evident reasons responsible for a problem, but, suffering is still viewed as a state of mind. Folk healers have evolved their own psychological theories about the functioning of human body and mind, which is hidden in their healing practices. The traditional therapies often result in symptomatic relief and better functioning of body. The diagnostic process in the traditional system of medicine seeks answers to the questions of what causes the disease and why it is affecting a particular person. The uniqueness of healing practices in the North-Western Himalayas is in considering the role of the '*Sacred*'. The entire belief system and myths of a community revolves around the concept of sacred & form the basis of magico-religious healing where the therapists activate strong psychic energies inside and outside the patient. The sacred may be evoked in many forms, such as the local versions of folk deities, ancestral spirits or at times evil-spirits. In all such therapies the physical and the metaphysical worlds overlap each other. The traditional healing process follows subsequent stages:

- Identification of the cause of violation of the customary order at physical and metaphysical levels;
- Removal or tackling with the cause hostile with the help of sorcerer, ancestral worship or asking for the forgiveness of deities or supernatural entities by making sacrifices or rituals to pacify their anger;
- Prescription of herbal medication or natural therapeutic procedures.

However, healing by folk healing is inclusive and has curative, protective and preventive elements. Depending on the cause of the disease, it is either natural or ritualistic, or both. A variety of treatment methods are recommended in folk medical therapeutics, for instance:

- Oral administration of medicated decoctions;

- Application of pastes/powdered medication on cuts or disease affected area;
- Inhalation of powdered preparation in the form of snuff/ smoke;
- Magico-religious or faith healing;
- Burning of incense to appease the deity; and
- Use of amulets to ward off evil spirits.

Communities living in theNorth-Western Himalayas believe that local deities and evil-spirits are as much part of this planet as they are of the metaphysical world and magico-religious or faith curing maintains a harmony between the two worlds. Herbal specialists or Herbalists, on the other hand, have acquired the knowledge of diagnosing and prescribing herbal medicines for day-to-day ailments as well as chronic diseases. The conceptual consequences of sickness, diagnosis and treatment are significant in understanding and managing sickness. The services of folk deities, supernatural healers and public health practitioners are sought for getting relief from various health ailments. These folk healers operate within a religious model, and hence there is no written material to confirm or support these traditions. The availability of different healers enables communities to switch from one type of health practitioner to another in search of the best. It seems the traditional herbal healers have inherited this art of healing from their forefathers which has a deep impact of the local culture. The herbal formulations prescribed by folk herbalists seem to have the impact of the ancient *Vedic* knowledge. Medicinal plants are used for preparing different herbal formulations. Different parts of medicinal plants-such as flower, fruit, root, latex, bark, stem and leaf are used.

Interviews with folk practitioners, for ascertaining the names of medicinal plants made it clear that there is a lot of ambiguity in nomenclature followed for naming the medicinal plants. In practice, folk practitioners across the region use different names for the same plant species. In old transcriptions, plant names have been mentioned with their medical functions, but no precise illustration has been made. The names of the medicinal plants disclosed by *Amchis* are in Tibetan language as described in the old scriptures. Healers are hesitant in disclosing their knowledge. It is this knowledge that provides them recognition in the society but they still believe that disclosing knowledge would lessen the effect of their medicine; hence they do not want to share it. This knowledge has been orally transferred from one generation to other. While diagnosing aliments, the folk herbalists extensively examine the patient physically including examination of pulse, complexion, eyes, tongue and skin. Thus, the traditional system of treatment prevalent in Himachal follows the basic approach of disease diagnosis mentioned in the ancient *Vedic* literature. Before starting any treatment, the healers examine the pulse, other signs and symptoms of a disease. Traditional Healers are repository of traditional knowledge especially for the utilization of plants for medicinal purposes. Many of the plants that are used by the *folk healers* find mention in ancient medicinal literature.

Customarily, the profession of a healer is valued as a matter of charity and, therefore, the fee of any kind for treatment is highly discouraged. This notion still persists in some parts of the state for some specific treatments; traditional healers do not accept anything from a person who undergoes treatment under them. The knowledge regarding the herbal use of plants is so deep rooted in the society that there are still number of women and men in the villages who know the healing properties of medicinal plants.

The loss of traditional knowledge regarding preparation of medicines is due to the decline in the number of healers coming forward to adopt this profession. In addition, the involvement of healers for identification of medicinal plants and preparing various formulations is declining rapidly. For future development of the region and country, the traditional system should be regarded and established as a valuable system. The herbal preparations used by the traditional healers must be scientifically tested and validated. The ongoing acceptance of *Ayurveda* in the West can be made useful to popularize it across the globe. The claimed curative properties of medicinal plants mentioned by various traditional healers must be clinically tested in order to establish their validity, and also to evolve new medical formulations. No doubt, the traditional medical system has survived for a very long time; its therapeutic value needs to be studied, researched and upgraded in the context of the present times, which would certainly add to the scope of the medical science as well as to the benefit of the humankind.

Appendix A
Dried Herbs

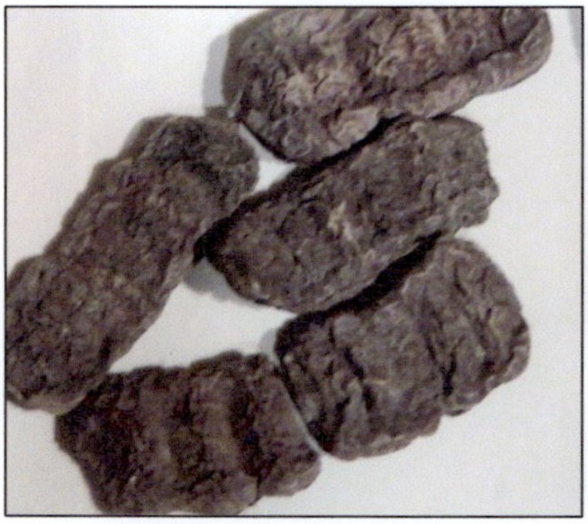

Acacia concinna (Dried Pod)

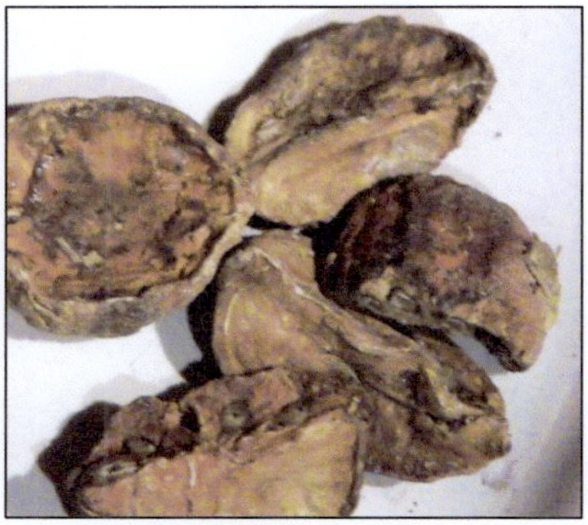

Aegle marmelos (Dried Fruit)

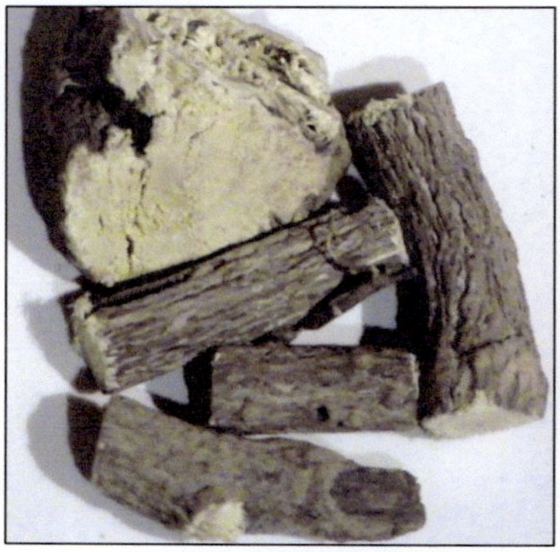

Glycerrhiza glabra (Dried Stem)

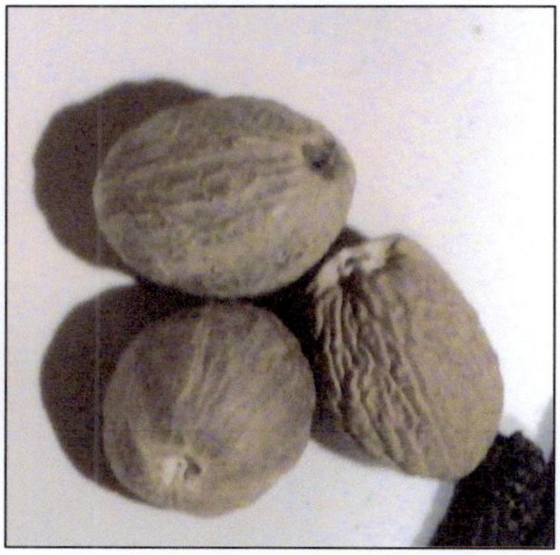

Myristica fragrans (Dried Fruit)

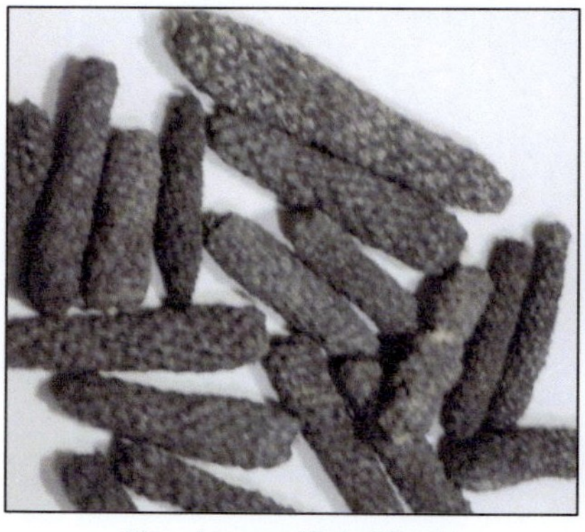

Piper longum (Dried Fruit)

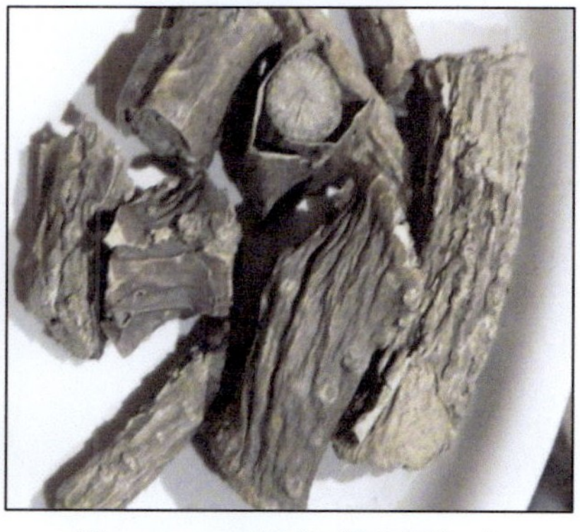

Tinospora cordifolia (Dried Stem)

P. Gupta et al., *Healing Traditions of the Northwestern Himalayas*,
SpringerBriefs in Environmental Science, DOI: 10.1007/978-81-322-1925-5,

Appendix B
Medicinal Plants

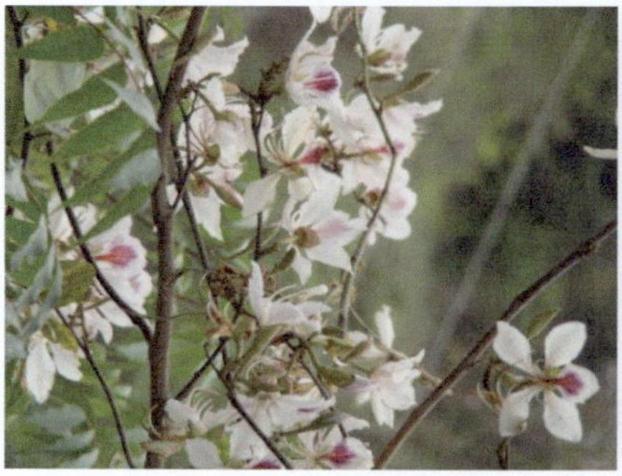

Bauhinia variegata

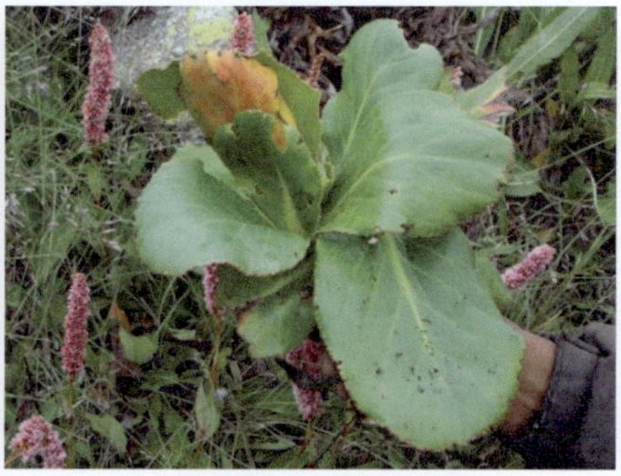

Bergenia ciliate

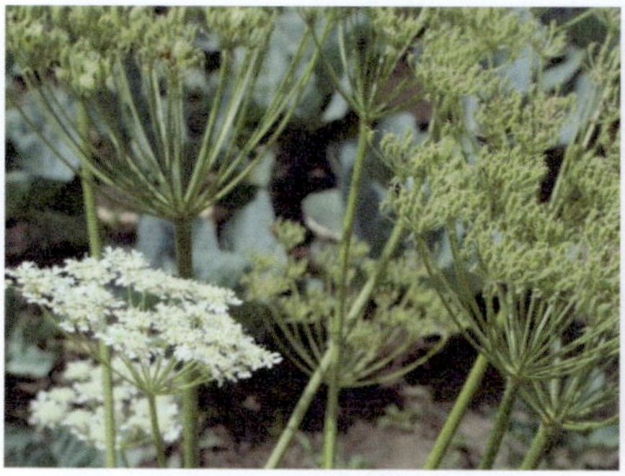

Heracleum lanatum

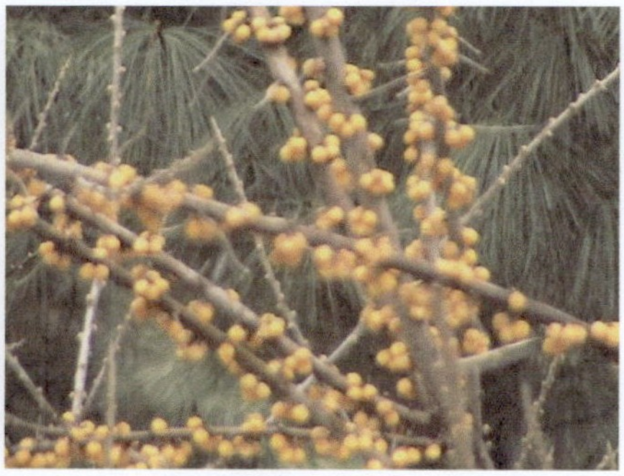

Hippophae rhamnoides

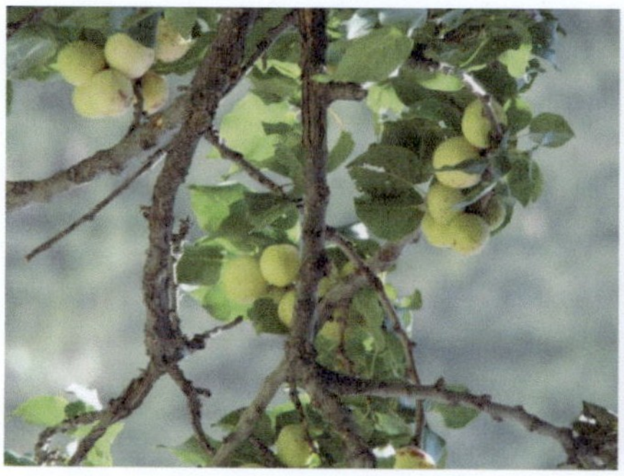

Prunus armeniaca

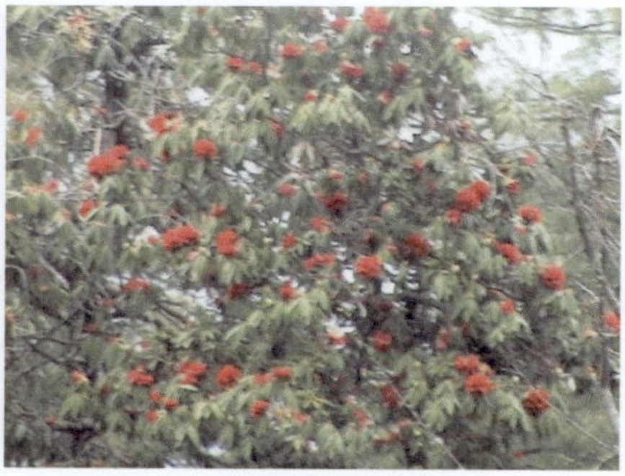

Rhododendron anthopogon

P. Gupta et al., *Healing Traditions of the Northwestern Himalayas*,
SpringerBriefs in Environmental Science, DOI: 10.1007/978-81-322-1925-5,

Appendix C
Medicinal Plants

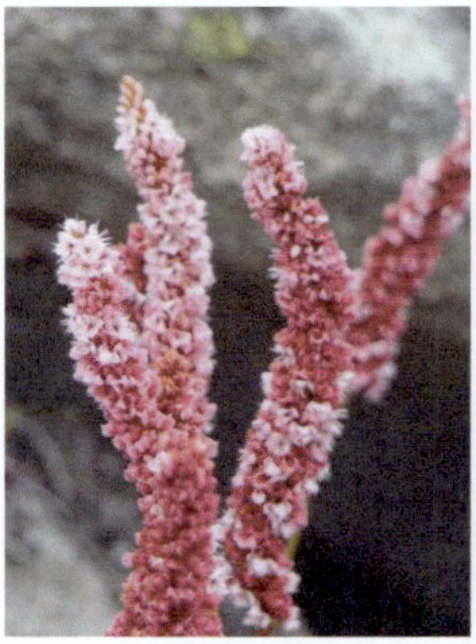

Bistorta affinis

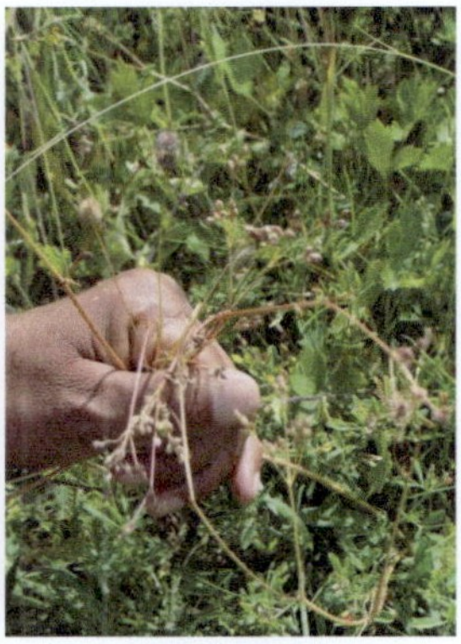

Bunium persicum

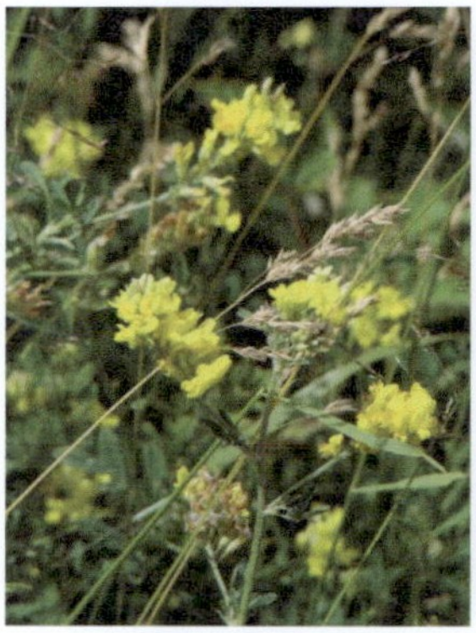

Medicago falcata

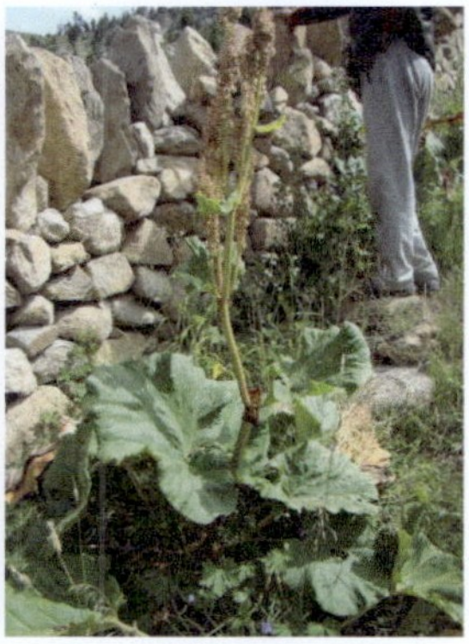

Rheum sp.

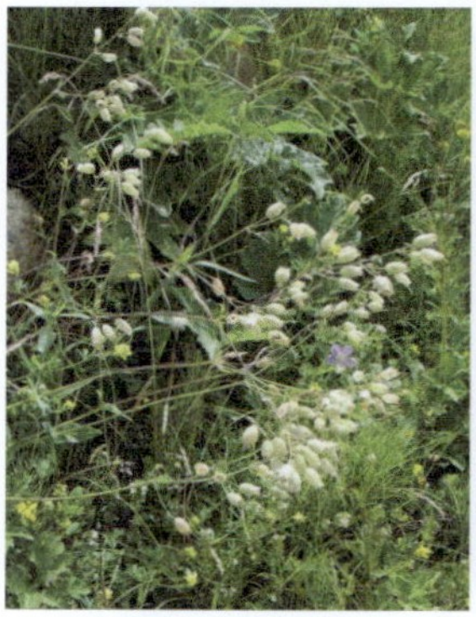

Silene cucubalus

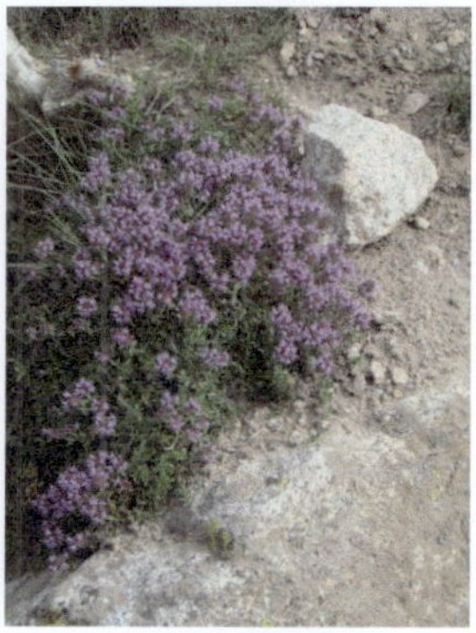

Thymus serpyllum

P. Gupta et al., *Healing Traditions of the Northwestern Himalayas*,
SpringerBriefs in Environmental Science, DOI: 10.1007/978-81-322-1925-5,

Bibliography

UNESCO. (2002). Best Practices using Indigenous Knowledge. Retrieved March 5, 2013, from http://www.unesco.org/most/Bpikpub2.pdf

P. Gupta et al., *Healing Traditions of the Northwestern Himalayas*,
SpringerBriefs in Environmental Science, DOI: 10.1007/978-81-322-1925-5,

About the Book

WHO defines Traditional medicine as wisdom, skills, and practices based on the theories, beliefs, and experiences indigenous to different cultures, used in prevention, diagnosis, improvement or treatment of physical and mental illness and maintenance of health. In some Asian and African countries, 80 % of the population depend on traditional medicine for primary health care. The book precisely uncovers indigenous health care traditions among Himalayan communities besides outlining the conventional and conservative interventions made by people for both physical and mental health at local level. The chapters cover a diverse range issues, including—People and knowledge systems, healing in ancient scriptures, concept of sacredness and faith healing, food as medicament, presumptions on disease, mystic healers as mediators between materialistic and metaphysical world for mental and physical health, ethno-botanical aspects of medicinal plants, collection and processing of herbs, traditional therapeutic procedures, indigenous Materia medica, etc. Besides, throwing light on people's perception on disease, healing concepts, and evolution of traditional systems of healing, it attempts to illustrate diverse therapeutic procedures followed by Himalayan healers and their significancein the socio-cultural life of Himalayan societies. Most of healing traditions on the verge of extinction were explored during the research and are presented in the monograph. The importance of safeguarding indigenous knowledge in context of cultural milieu of Himalayan region is crucial. From a socio-cultural standpoint, it examines specific interventions made by traditional Himalayan societies for treatment and health care access. This book will be an invaluable resource for researchers across many disciplines, like medical anthropology, biology, ethnobiology, ecology, community health, health behavior, psychotherapy, and Himalayan studies.

P. Gupta et al., *Healing Traditions of the Northwestern Himalayas*,
SpringerBriefs in Environmental Science, DOI: 10.1007/978-81-322-1925-5,

MIX
Papier aus verantwortungsvollen Quellen
Paper from responsible sources
FSC® C105338

If you have any concerns about our products,
you can contact us on
ProductSafety@springernature.com

In case Publisher is established outside the EU,
the EU authorized representative is:
Springer Nature Customer Service Center GmbH
Europaplatz 3, 69115 Heidelberg, Germany

Printed by Libri Plureos GmbH
in Hamburg, Germany